NURSING 1

MULTIPLE CHOICE QUESTIO

NURSING 1

MULTIPLE CHOICE QUESTIONS

D. MIDDLETON
SRN, RNT
Tutor, Charles Frears School
of Nursing, Leicester

Blackwell Scientific Publications
OXFORD LONDON EDINBURGH
BOSTON PALO ALTO MELBOURNE

Editorial offices:
Osney Mead, Oxford OX2 0EL
8 John Street, London WC1N 2ES
23 Ainslie Place, Edinburgh, EH3 6AJ
52 Beacon Street, Boston
Massachusetts 02108, USA
667 Lytton Avenue, Palo Alto
California 94301, USA
107 Barry Street, Carlton
Victoria 3053, Australia

First published 1983
Reprinted 1986

Filmset at the Alden Press, Oxford.
Printed and bound in Great Britain
by Billing and Sons Ltd, Worcester

DISTRIBUTORS

USA
Year Book Medical Publishers
35 East Wacker Drive
Chicago, Illinois 60601

Canada
The C.V. Mosby Company
5240 Finch Avenue East,
Scarborough, Ontario

Australia
Blackwell Scientific Publications
(Australia) Pty Ltd
107 Barry Street
Carlton, Victoria 3053

British Library
Cataloguing in Publication Data

Middleton, D.
Nursing.
1: Multiple choice questions.
1. Nursing—Problems, exercises, etc.
I. Title
610.73'076 RT55

ISBN 0-632-00959-4

Contents

Orthopaedic Case Histories

Geriatric Case Histories

ANSWERS

Preface

Although it can stand on its own merit, this book is intended as a companion text to *Nursing 1*, which is a basic nursing text outlining nursing care and its application to a variety of illnesses which the nurse learner is likely to meet during the first 18 months of a general training.

There are four distinct parts to the book, 40 case histories, each followed by 10 multiple choice type questions, making a total of 400 questions. For each case study and 10 questions there is an answer sheet.

The case studies have been selected carefully because of their frequency in the average nurse's common core experience. They can also be used as a resource on which to build hypothetical nursing care plans based on the nursing process, such an activity of itself will consolidate theoretical knowledge.

Each case study is followed by 10 multiple choice type questions. It requires the learner to read the stem of each question carefully being certain of selecting key phrases or words which will direct their attention to the correct option. There is only one correct option to each question, the other three options are intended as distractors. A distractor can be blatantly untrue or very near the truth, and may require the learner to refer back to the case study for clarification of the answer. On average a learner should obtain a score of between 4 to 7 for each test after a reasonable period of study. The questions have been designed to discriminate equally between a wide variety of ability in the nurse learner population.

The answer sheets should qualify the reasons and rationale for the correct answer, more importantly they should be used in conjunction with the case studies to obtain deeper insights into the illness being studied.

This type of examination, that is, questions based on a case study is shortly to be introduced by the statutory examination body for England and Wales, and the author hopes this book will make a contribution in preparing nurse learners for their final examination.

Acknowledgements

I wish to thank the pupil and student nurses of the Charles Frears School of Nursing for their cooperation and suggestions during the testing of these case studies. From their work the author is quite confident that the text is valid for nurse learners during their first 18 months of training.

May I also extend my appreciation to Miss J. Turton SRN, SCM, RNT, Senior Nurse Tutor Mansfield School of Nursing, for reviewing this manuscript and giving many useful suggestions which sharpened the text and made the compilation of the text an enjoyable task.

Medical Case Histories

1 Pernicious Anaemia

PATIENT'S PROFILE

Mrs Drobney has pernicious anaemia. During her hospital stay she has received a deep intramuscular injection of iron–dextran (Imferon) 50 mg, a transfusion of 2 units of packed erythrocytes and has commenced on a course of hydroxocobalamin (Neo-Cytamen) on alternate days for 2 weeks.

In addition to basic nursing care Mrs Drobney has been encouraged to eat a high protein diet and to rest. Observations in the early phase of therapy included recording her pulse, blood pressure, and fluid intake and output. Mrs Drobney's red cell count, haemoglobin and packed cell volume are now within normal limits and she is due for discharge from hospital in a few days time.

1.1 **When taking Mrs Drobney's observations in the early phase of therapy the nurse notices that the pulse is rapid and the blood pressure low. Both these symptoms are probably due to:**

a physical exhaustion
b peripheral anoxia
c hypotension
d transfusion of packed cells

1.2 **Hydroxocobalamin has been prescribed to Mrs Drobney because she lacks:**

a extrinsic factor
b gastrin hormone
c intrinsic factor
d hydrochloric acid

1.3 Injections of iron–dextran are given deeply into the muscle using the Z method. This technique is recommended because iron–dextran can:

a be very painful
b easily reflux along the needle track
c stain the superficial tissues
d readily damage a nerve fibre

1.4 Hydroxocobalamin is normally prescribed in amounts of 1000 μg. This dose is equivalent to one:

a milligram
b microgram
c nanogram
d picogram

1.5 Hydroxocobalamin's equivalent in normal diet is vitamin:

a B_1
b B_2
c B_6
d B_{12}

1.6 The packed cells transfused to Mrs Drobney contain:

a erythroblasts
b erythrocytes
c leucocytes
d thrombocytes

1.7 One investigation which may have confirmed the diagnosis of pernicious anaemia is the:

a Snellen's test
b Schilling test
c Schiller's test
d Schlesinger's test

1.8 The most important piece of advice that Mrs Drobney should be given before her discharge from hospital is that she:

a will require maintenance therapy for life
b needs to continue taking a high-protein diet
c should continue to take specific rest periods during the day
d should aim at maintaining constant body weight

1.9 **During Mrs Drobney's hospital stay the doctor gave her a complete neurological examination to exclude the possibility of:**

a subacute optical neuritis
b subacute disseminated sclerosis
c subacute degeneration of the spinal cord
d bilateral degeneration of the thoracic nerves

1.10 **The symptoms of pernicious anaemia tend to be slow and insidious. This is because large reserves of cyanocobalamin are stored in the:**

a bone
b pancreas
c liver
d spleen

2 Chronic Bronchitis

PATIENT'S PROFILE

Mr James has suffered from chronic bronchitis for several years, but is now to be admitted into hospital because of a severe dyspnoeic attack brought about by an acute respiratory infection. He is obviously struggling for breath, relying on oral respiration. His skin is very cyanosed and there is evidence of pitting oedema of the ankles. The medical instructions regarding the treatment of Mr James include:

bedrest
a specimen of sputum for pathology
humidified oxygen 4 litres per minute at 28% concentration
frusemide (Lasix) 40 mg orally once daily
2 aminophylline suppositories each evening
tetracycline 250 mg every four hours.
encouragement to take fluids orally

2.1 **The requested specimen of sputum may help to:**

a determine the degree of the acute infection
b identify the causative organism of the infection
c assess the volume of bronchial secretions
d measure the viscosity of the bronchial secretions

2.2 **As the oxygen is humidified this will help Mr James because it primarily:**

a prevents the bronchial mucosa from becoming dry
b reduces the viscosity of the bronchial secretions
c promotes gaseous exchange at the alveoli
d allows for greater expansion of the lobes of the lungs

2.3 **A broad spectrum antibiotic such as tetracycline has been prescribed because it is effective against:**

a bacteria and viruses
b specific respiratory bacteria
c several species of bacteria
d specific respiratory viruses

2.4 **Frusemide encourages a diuresis by acting within the kidney on the:**

a loop of Henle, collecting duct and glomerulus
b distal tubule, proximal tubule and loop of Henle
c proximal tubule, glomerulus and collecting duct
d glomerulus, loop of Henle and proximal tubule

2.5 **The aminophylline suppositories administered to Mr James during the evening will improve his respiration by causing:**

a relaxation of the alveoli
b vasodilation of the pulmonary blood supply
c relaxation of the bronchial smooth muscle
d inhibition of the nerve supply to the diaphragm

2.6 **Mr James should be encouraged to drink at least 2 litres of fluids per day because this:**

a eliminates the need for intravenous therapy
b prevents the tendency to dehydration
c reduces the need to give oral toilet
d compensates for the diuretic effect of frusemide

2.7 Cyanosis at the peripheries indicates that there is:

a evidence of peripheral oedema
b vasoconstriction of the peripheral vessels
c shallow but rapid respirations
d an increase of carbon dioxide in the lungs

2.8 The mucosa of the buccal cavity will tend to be:

a moist and healthy
b dry and prone to infection
c unaffected by the dyspnoea
d dirty and infected

2.9 Which of the following defines the vital capacity of the lungs, the:

a maximum volume of air expired after a maximal inhalation
b residual volume of air remaining in the lungs after a maximal exhalation
c average volume of air inhaled after a normal exhalation of air
d difference between the air volume of a minimal and maximal respiration

2.10 After Mr James has recovered from his dyspnoeic attack his vital capacity of air is more likely to be:

a the same as it was prior to the acute infection
b much improved on how it was prior to his dyspnoea
c reduced to that prior to his hospital admission
d much improved on that prior to the acute infection

3 Myocardial Infarction

PATIENT'S PROFILE

Forty-eight hours after suffering from a myocardial infarction Mr O'Brien is being transferred from the coronary unit to a medical ward on the following regimen:

bedrest until further instructions

heparin 5000 units by slow infusion which will conclude after 6 hours

Anticoagulant with interactions similar to warfarin

phenindione (Dindevan) 25 mg at 10.00 and 18.00 hours

daily prothrombin time

digoxin (Lanoxin) 0.25 mg daily at 10.00 hours

diamorphine hydrochloride (Heroin) 10 mg once only if required for pain

prochlorperazine (Stemetil) 12.5 mg as necessary

clear fluids only

cardiac monitoring until otherwise instructed

Mrs O'Brien has been staying in the hospital since her husband's admission and cannot be persuaded to go home.

It is known that Mr O'Brien smokes rather heavily and works very hard as a sales manager for a furnishing company. For several years now Mr O'Brien has tended towards obesity.

3.1 **Mr O'Brien will remain on bedrest and be dependent on nursing skills until:**

a his blood pressure and pulse stay within normal limits for at least 24 hours
b the prothrombin time remains stable between 15 and 25 seconds for 48 hours
c the cardiac rhythm remains normal for at least 24 hours
d the raised serum cardiac enzymes return to normal limits

3.2 **Digoxin improves the cardiac output by strengthening the contractions of the ventricles. An essential observation before its administration is to:**

a record the blood pressure
b assess the pulse volume
c assess the fluid intake and output
d assess the apex beat or the radial pulse

3.3 **During a routine testing of Mr O'Brien's urine the nurse observes a trace reaction of blood on the chemical reagent strip. Which drug is likely to have caused a mild haematuria:**

a digoxin
b diamorphine
c phenindione
d prochlorperazine

3·4 As the nurse administers the phenindione to Mr O'Brien which antidote should the nurse ensure is also available:

a protamine sulphate
b phytomenadione (vitamin K)
c hydroxocobalamin (vitamin B_{12})
d adrenaline

3·5 Mr O'Brien asks the nurse what exactly a myocardial infarction is; the nurse's answer should describe that it is:

a atheroma of the coronary arteries
d ischaemia of the heart muscle
c necrosis of the heart muscle
d thrombosis of a coronary artery

3·6 After Mr O'Brien has been given an injection of diamorphine 10 mg his wife asks the nurse if her husband will live after suffering such severe pain. The most professional reply to such a question would be for the nurse to consider saying:

a 'The physician has everything under control, so please don't worry.'
b 'I really don't know, you had better see the physician.'
c 'His condition is very serious, please remain on hand to see the doctor.'
d 'Of course he will, everything possible is being done to pull him through.'

3·7 Several hours after his admission to the ward Mr O'Brien complains of chest pain which is radiating down his left arm. Should the nurse immediately:

a check both radial pulses and the blood pressure
b inform the most senior colleague on duty
c reassure Mr O'Brien that the pain will recede eventually
d prepare to give an intramuscular injection of diamorphine

3.8 **Mr O'Brien will have to stop smoking and reduce the amount of arduous work he would normally do. Who is best placed to ensure this advice is respected:**

a the physician

b the senior nurse caring for Mr O'Brien

c Mrs O'Brien

d Mr O'Brien's employer

3.9 **To help Mr O'Brien reduce his weight the nurse could introduce both Mr and Mrs O'Brien to the advantages of a:**

a cholesterol-free diet

b calorie-controlled diet

c carbohydrate-reducing diet

d control of dietary fats

3.10 **After being discharged from hospital Mr O'Brien is to continue having his prothrombin time measured twice a week. This test is done to:**

a warn of the tendency to minor haemorrhages

b determine the correct dosage of anticoagulants

c determine the correct dosage of digoxin

d assess the clotting time of blood

4 Congestive Cardiac Failure

PATIENT'S PROFILE

Mrs Morgan, a middle-aged lady, is an emergency admission who has severe dyspnoea and a marked oedema of both lower limbs and her abdomen. Her provisional diagnosis is stated as congestive cardiac failure and her medical regimen is prescribed as:

bedrest until both oedema and dyspnoea resolve
nursed on a cardiac bed
digoxin (Lanoxin) 0.25 mg at 10.00 and 18.00 hours
frusemide (Lasix) 40 mg at 10.00 hours daily
potassium chloride 1200 mg at 18.00 hours daily
diet as preferred but fluid balance charted

4.1 A provisional diagnosis of congestive cardiac failure should tell the nurse that Mrs Morgan has:

a an inadequate ventricular output
b pulmonary emphysema
c a blood pressure which is extremely high
d an incompetent aortic valve

4.2 Mrs Morgan's therapy should create a diuresis. The most accurate method of estimating if this is occurring is to:

a record her fluid intake and output
b record her weight every day
c measure the skinfold thickness of her upper arm each day
d measure and record the abdominal girth each day

4.3 The prime purpose of giving Mrs Morgan potassium chloride (Slow K) at 18.00 hours each day is:

a that in combination with the frusemide it will cause a diuresis
b to counteract the possibility of a hypokalaemia
c that in combination with digoxin it will correct cardiac arrhythmia
d to counteract the possibility of a hyperkalaemia

4.4 Prior to giving Mrs Morgan her digoxin the nurse checks the radial pulse and records it as being 48 beats per minute. Should the nurse:

a give Mrs Morgan her digoxin and inform the physician of the bradycardia
b check the apex beat and the blood pressure
c omit the drug and advise a senior colleague of Mrs Morgan's bradycardia
d advise Mrs Morgan she will have to wait for her medication

4.5 The Lasix has been prescribed for 10.00 hours. This is recommended because:

a the effect of Lasix is mediated when combined with potassium chloride
b the effect of digoxin should correspond with the Lasix
c the rapid effect of Lasix gives a diuresis during the day
d the delayed effect of Lasix defers a diuresis until the evening

4.6 **To help relieve the oedema the nurse could suggest to Mrs Morgan that one of the following be limited in her preferred diet:**

a potassium
b sodium chloride
c glucose and other sugars
d animal fats and cholesterol

4.7 **Mrs Morgan complains to nurse that she feels nauseated most of the time. The nurse could explain in simple terms that this is most probably due to:**

a cardiopulmonary oedema
b gastrointestinal oedema
c a side effect of one of her drugs
d her breathlessness and light diet

4.8 **One of the contributory factors to Mrs Morgan's oedema is that the blood pressure at the:**

a venules exceeds that of the osmotic pressure
b arterioles exceeds that of the osmotic pressure
c veins exceeds the arterial pressure
d arteries exceeds that of the veins

4.9 **Until Mrs Morgan's oedema is effectively relieved and the dyspnoea less marked she should be nursed sitting upright:**

a with the head of the bed elevated
b with the foot of the bed elevated
c in an armchair with both legs elevated on a footstool
d with the mattress at a horizontal level

4.10 **Congestive cardiac failure commonly progresses to:**

a myocardial infarction
b pulmonary embolism
c peripheral hypertension and cerebral thrombosis
d left ventricular failure and oedema

5 Asthma

PATIENT'S PROFILE

On his first day at playschool Darren was naturally shy and reluctant to let go of his mother's hand when she tried to leave the playroom. Only with a great deal of coaxing did Darren eventually leave his mother and go to look at the small animals in the 'pets' corner. The playleader pointed out the two rabbits in a cage, noting Darren's animation she encouraged him to open the cage and stroke one of them.

Within a few minutes Darren started to breathe rather noisily and was soon gasping for air. With a terrified scream he fell to the floor still struggling for breath and rapidly becoming blue around his lips and ears. For several seconds the playleader was dumbfounded but, quickly recovering her wits, she rushed to the telephone and summoned an ambulance and then made a second call to Darren's home advising the relatives that Darren's mother should come to the local hospital immediately. Until the ambulance arrived she made Darren as comfortable as possible.

On arrival at the accident and emergency department Darren was almost comatose, he still gasped for air and was wheezing. The doctor immediately administered adrenaline 1–1000 and aminophylline 0.125 g by subcutaneous injection with an immediate beneficial effect. There was a slight improvement in Darren's inspiratory breathing but he continued to wheeze on expiration. Although he was more alert, Darren remained visibly terrified. When Darren's mother arrived he immediately relaxed and although agitated she was able to clarify that Darren had never had such an attack before, nor could she remember any of the immediate or extended family having experienced any allergic or atopic problems.

Giving a diagnosis of asthma the doctor advised admission to hospital on the following regimen:

normal saline 0.9% 500 ml intravenously for 12 hours
continuous oxygen therapy at 28% concentration 6–8 litres per minute nebulized with salbutamol via an inspiron mask
peak flow readings every 4 hours
chlorpromazine (Largactil) 25 mg three times daily
chest physiotherapy twice daily

On admission Darren's observations were recorded as being:

pulse 140 beats per minute, barely perceptible

NB inspiron = The act of drawing in the breath.

respirations 40 per minute
blood pressure 13/7 kPa (90/50 mmHg)

The doctor asked to be notified immediately if there was any discernible deterioration in Darren's condition and for the observations to be recorded every 30 minutes.

5.1 **At the time of the asthmatic attack the playgroup leader could make Darren more comfortable by:**

a placing him in the lateral position resting his head on a pillow
b resting him in the prone position across her knee while she sat on a chair
c sitting him upright supporting his bodyweight in her arms
d wrapping him in a warm blanket and placing him in the supine position on the floor

5.2 **The most vital observation which indicates if there is any deterioration in Darren's condition after his admission to the ward is:**

a a pulse rate exceeding 100 beats per minute
b severe peripheral cyanosis
c a fixed shoulder girdle during inspiration
d increasing drowsiness

5.3 **The respiratory changes from which Darren is suffering result in the:**

a collapse in the alveoli
b constriction of the bronchiolar lumen
c spasm of the intercostal muscles
d overt stimulation of the phrenic nerve

5.4 **The altered respiratory cycle has most probably been initiated by:**

a intrinsic factors
b emotional responses
c extrinsic factors
d genetic predisposition

5.5 Darren is 100 cm in height; the expected average peak flow readings from a boy of his age would be:

a 400 litres of air per minute
b 200 litres of oxygen per minute
c 200 litres of air per minute
d 400 litres of oxygen per minute

5.6 Several hours after his initial asthmatic attack Darren experienced difficulty clearing the respiratory tract of thick tenacious mucus. The best non-mechanical method of aiding expectoration in this instance would be by:

a oropharnygeal suction
b broad spectrum antibiotics
c bronchial dilators
d chest physiotherapy

5.7 The most effective method of administering Darren's prescribed oxygen therapy is by using a:

a perforated oxygen mask
b sealed oxygen mask
c nasal catheters
d oxygen tent

5.8 Darren's condition responds to the prescribed regimen but he continues, however, to be emotionally agitated. Such distress may respond to:

a aminophylline
b adrenaline
c salbutamol
d chlorpromazine

5.9 The nurse could advise Darren's mother that further attacks could be prevented by:

a never leaving Darren alone in a strange environment
b employing domestic cleaning methods which control dust levels in the home
c never losing her temper in front of her son
d limiting the family contact with domestic pets

5.10 **Prior to discharge from hospital Darren is prescribed an Intal inhaler (sodium cromoglycate). This drug acts by:**

a limiting the effect of circulating toxic amines
b destroying the effect of circulating histamine
c preventing the release of excessive histamine
d desensitizing the tissues to the effect of toxic amines

6 Deep Vein Thrombosis and Pulmonary Embolus

PATIENT'S PROFILE

Michael, aged 36, works as a car mechanic in a small garage. He is a happily married man whose wife works as a part-time hairdresser which gives her plenty of time to care for their 4-year-old son. Michael does not smoke but enjoys four or five pints of beer each weekend.

For several weeks Michael had been troubled by pain in the right calf muscle and had some swelling around the ankle. His general practitioner was reassuring describing the pain as 'cramp' and prescribed ibuprofen (Brufen) 600 mg to be taken three times a day for seven days. Although the ankle swelling resolved, the cramp-like pain remained a constant problem. On a second visit to his doctor Michael was again reassured and was given a second prescription of ibuprofen at a reduced dose, i.e., 300 mg for a further week.

Two days before going abroad on a family holiday Michael suffered an acute pain over the right chest wall on inspiration. The emergency doctor on call visited Michael at his home and advised admission to hospital. He told Michael that he had a blood clot in the right leg and pleurisy both requiring hospital treatment.

After an extensive examination the admitting physician stated the diagnosis as deep vein thrombosis and pulmonary embolism. He prescribed:

bedrest for 72 hours
supportive bandaging for both limbs
heparin 20000 units every 6 hours via an intravenous pump for 72 hours
warfarin 5 mg once daily at 18.00 hours

After his admission the following investigations were done on Michael:

lung scan
chest X-ray
venogram
daily prothrombin time

The observations recorded by the admitting nurse showed that Michael's temperature was normal, the radial pulse was 96 beats per minute, his blood pressure was 18/12 kPa (136/90 mmHg), respirations 20 per minute and a routine urinalysis proved negative. Michael's weight was 95 kilograms and his height 175 centimetres.

6.1 Ibuprofen is a drug which can be grouped as an:

a analgesic
b anti-inflammatory agent
c muscle relaxant
d hypotensive agent

6.2 Given Michael's height and weight it would be correct to assume that he is

a underweight
b normal weight
c overweight
d obese

6.3 The desired effect of the administered heparin is to:

a prevent the thrombosis from enlarging
b liquefy the fibrin within the thrombus and embolus
c boost the production of naturally occurring heparin
d prolong the bleeding time of blood

6.4 Which of the following would prolong the effect of heparin and should not be given to Michael:

a protamine sulphate
b acetylsalicylic acid
c codeine phosphate
d vitamin K_1

6.5 The nurse applied TED stockings to Michael's lower limbs. The purpose of elasticated hosiery is to:

a counteract the tendency of ankle oedema
b compress the deep veins of the lower limbs
c compress the superficial veins of the legs
d relieve the persistent cramp-like pain

6.6 Michael was nursed in the recumbent position. Believing it would be more comfortable he placed one of his pillows under his knees. The nurse removed this pillow explaining to Michael that it was dangerous because it:

a compressed the popliteal artery
b caused stiffness of the knee cartilages
c impeded bloodflow to both legs
d compressed the popliteal veins

6.7 The pulmonary emboli was a fragment of the thrombosis. This fragment detached itself and travelled to the right lung via the:

a pulmonary veins
b iliac and hepatic veins
c inferior vena cava
d superior vena cava

6.8 Which one factor may have contributed to Michael's deep vein thrombosis? His:

a idiopathy
b alcohol intake
c hypertension
d body weight

6.9 In preparing Michael for the venogram the nurse should advise him that:

a there is no particular preparation for this non-invasive X-ray
b apart from being starved for 6 hours there is no other preparation
c he will be prepared for general anaesthesia
d the injection of dye may cause a burning sensation

6.10 Michael made a good recovery, and 11 days later he was discharged but had to continue to take warfarin 5 mg daily until his next outpatient appointment in 10 days' time. Michael should be advised to:

a contact his general practitioner to arrange for regular prothrombin time tests
b continue to take prolonged rest periods during the day
c return to work as soon as possible
d arrange to take the family holiday in a few months' time

7 Hypertension

PATIENT'S PROFILE

Mr Arnold is a 57-year-old married man who is the managing director of a busy engineering firm. Recently he has become increasingly breathless, suffers occasionally from blinding headaches and describes himself as feeling rather tense. His general practitioner is concerned with Mr Arnold's rather high blood pressure reading of 32/16 kPa (220/110 mmHg). He advises Mr Arnold that further hospital investigations would be to his advantage and also provide the means of giving him a rest from his irregular work hours. The admitting physician notes that Mr Arnold smokes about 30 cigarettes a day and is 18 kg overweight. The medical instructions are listed as:

phenobarbitone 30 mg twice daily at 10.00 and 18.00 hours
methyldopa (Aldomet) 250 mg twice daily at 10.00 and 18.00 hours
frusemide (Lasix) 20 mg twice daily at 10.00 and 18.00 hours
an electrocardiogram
24-hour urine collection for vanillylmandelic acid (VMA)
blood pressure recordings every 4 hours during the daytime

7.1 The combination of drugs prescribed for Mr Arnold can be grouped as follows:

a analgesics, tranquillizers, and hypotensive agents
b sedatives, diuretics and hypotensive agents
c diuretics, analgesics and hypotensive agents
d vasoconstrictors, diuretics and analgesics

7.2 **Which of the following factors in Mr Arnold's background are mostly likely to be contributing to his hypertension:**

a alcohol, working hours and blood pressure

b obesity, alcohol and smoking

c anxiety, obesity and smoking

d alcohol, high blood pressure and headaches

7.3 **Mr Arnold's electrocardiogram shows a distortion of the T wave. This may imply an abnormality in:**

a ventricular contraction

b auricular relaxation

c ventricular relaxation

d auricular contraction

7.4 **While taking Mr Arnold's blood pressure the nurse is detecting the diastolic reading which indicates the pressure occurring during:**

a ventricular contraction

b auricular and ventricular relaxation

c ventricular relaxation

d auricular and ventricular contraction

7.5 **Mr Arnold's specimen collection of urine should commence and conclude from 08.00–08.00 hours. The nurse should:**

a discard the commencing specimen and save all other urine passed in the 24-hour period

b save all the urine except the concluding specimen which is discarded

c discard both commencing and concluding specimens and save all other urine

d save all the urine passed in the 24-hour period

7.6 **The prime action of methyldopa is to oppose the constriction of the:**

a arterioles

b arteries

c venules

d veins

7.7 Forty-eight hours after his prescribed therapy the nurse notes that Mr Arnold has lost 3 kg of bodyweight. This implies that:

a rest and sedation are reducing the body's metabolic rate
b urinary secretion and excretion have increased
c the dietary protein should be increased
d his hypertension is responding to therapy

7.8 After 4 days of therapy Mr Arnold feels much better and considers himself cured. He tells the nurse he would like to go home and if necessary discharge himself. The nurse should:

a ensure that Mr Arnold signs a self-discharge form before leaving the hospital
b contact Mrs Arnold advising her that her husband is on his way home
c persuade Mr Arnold that his therapy is long-term and he should stay in hospital
d request that Mr Arnold consult his physician before leaving the hospital

7.9 Three contributing factors to the maintenance of normal blood pressure are cardiac output and:

a blood viscosity and arteriole constriction
b arterial and venous constriction
c capillary constriction and blood viscosity
d arterial constriction and plasma protein

7.10 An important aspect of advice which should be given by the dietician and reinforced by the nurse concerning Mr Arnold's diet after hospital discharge is to:

a eliminate table salt and control his cholesterol intake
b control both carbohydrate and protein intake
c control his calorie intake and evaluate methods of cooking
d replace all saturated and unsaturated fats

8 Mature Onset Diabetes

PATIENT'S PROFILE

Mrs Doris Arundel, aged 50, has been referred to the hospital diabetic clinic by her general practitioner. Doris has been visiting her GP concerning an irritating itching of her skin and also of the vulva. On questioning it is noted that Doris is overweight for her age and stature. On routine urinalysis she has a glycosuria of 1%. No one else in Mrs Arundel's immediate or extended family has a history of diabetes and her three teenage sons are very healthy. The physician decides to admit Doris and asks for:

4 hourly urinalysis for glycosuria
4 hourly blood pressure reading
a glucose tolerance on the following day
1000 calorie diet (4.2 kiloJoules)

The physician subsequently orders chlorpropamide (Diabinese) 250 mg once daily.

8.1 An alternative name for the itching of the skin is:

- **a** petechia
- **b** pruritus
- **c** psoriasis
- **d** polydipsia

8.2 When preparing Mrs Arundel for her glucose tolerance test the nurse would be correct in advising her that:

- **a** she will have an injection of insulin prior to blood being taken for the test
- **b** she will need to empty her bladder before blood is taken for the test
- **c** she will remain fasting overnight prior to the first blood sample being taken
- **d** she must remain on bedrest during the whole period of the test

8.3 Mrs Arundel will be given a set amount of glucose to drink during the test. The test results will show whether:

a she can stabilize her blood sugar within normal limits
b the liver can convert glucose to glycogen
c the intestine can absorb glucose to within normal limits
d the pancreas can excrete sufficient insulin

8.4 During the glucose tolerance test the blood glucose level can be expected to peak within:

a 1–2 mmol per litre (18–36 mg per 100 ml)
b 3–5 mmol per litre (55–90 mg per 100 ml)
c 7–9 mmol per litre (125–180 mg per 100 ml)
d 10–12 mmol per litre (185–200 mg per 100 ml)

8.5 When Mrs Arundel is being taught for the first time how to test her urine she asks the nurse what is precisely meant by a 1% reaction. The nurse could correctly answer that this indicates there is:

a 1 g of glucose in every 100 ml of urine excreted
b 10 g of glucose in every 100 ml of urine excreted
c 1 g of glucose in every 10 ml of urine excreted
d 10 g of glucose in every 10 ml of urine excreted

8.6 Mrs Arundel would be regarded as being obese if her weight was above the recommended ideal by:

a 5%
b 10%
c 15%
d 20%

8.7 When checking Mrs Arundel's blood pressure chart the nurse observes that the systolic pressure reading is variable, never falling below 17 kPa (120 mmHg) but rising to as high as 22 kPa (170 mmHg) occasionally. Such changes may indicate to the nurse that:

a the 1000 calorie diet is far too generous and should be reduced
b the renal threshold for glucose is remaining constant
c there is evidence of heart failure
d the intima of the arteries is in some way damaged

8.8 In discussing the chlorpropamide with Mrs Arundel the nurse should stress the importance to her of one effect of the drug which is:

a peripheral swelling due to oedema
b alcohol intolerance
c vertigo and headaches
d hypoglycaemia

8.9 The major long-term complication of mature onset diabetes could be minimized if the nurse stresses to Mrs Arundel to take care and:

a ensure that she has chlorpropamide each day at the prescribed times
b have an annual check up in addition to her hospital visits
c contact the Diabetic Association for further counselling about diabetes
d ensure that both hosiery and footwear are correctly fitted and comfortable

8.10 The eldest of Mrs Arundel's sons is about to be married and asks the nurse what are the possibilities of his mother's condition being genetic. The best reply to this query is that mature onset diabetes:

a has a 1 in 4 chance of being inherited
b tends to occur in families but is not genetic
c occurs spontaneously and the cause is not known
d is due to virus infection and is not inherited

9 Juvenile Onset Diabetes

PATIENT'S PROFILE

Michael, who is 15 years old, has had a medical history of diabetes since he was seven. In the last few days he has been suffering from a very severe attack of influenza, pyrexia and having several episodes of vomiting. His general practitioner has altered his existing regimen of 8 units of insulin zinc suspension daily to 12 units of soluble insulin twice daily. This, however, has not brought Michael's glycosuria and high blood sugar under reasonable control. As a last resort the doctor has asked the consultant to visit Michael for a specialist opinion. The consultant decides that Michael requires hospitalization to control his diabetes during his illness of influenza, and admits him giving the following instructions:

4 hourly urinalysis for glucose and ketones
soluble insulin 8 units at 08.00 and 18.00 hours
180 g carbohydrate diet
blood sugar estimation every 4 hours (Dextrostix)

9.1 **The glycosuria will result in a raised:**
- a metabolic rate
- b specific gravity
- c blood pressure
- d pulse rate

9.2 **After receiving his first insulin injection Michael complains of feeling unwell. He tells nurse that his vision is blurred and his skin is cold and clammy. The nurse should immediately prepare:**
- a for the administration of intravenous dextrose
- b to give 20 g glucose in water
- c to collect and test a specimen of urine
- d the equipment necessary to collect a blood specimen

9.3 **The insulin administered to Michael would normally have the expected effect of:**
- a delaying the glucose from entering the cells
- b actively promoting secretion from the pancreatic alpha cells
- c allowing the cells to utilize glucose
- d actively promoting secretion from the pancreatic beta cells

9.4 **The ward sister or charge nurse instructs the nurse to observe Michael for any evidence of hyperglycaemia. The most likely sign that hyperglycaemia may occur is if the:**
- a skin becomes pale and moist
- b pulse becomes full and irregular
- c skin becomes dry and inelastic
- d abdomen becomes painful

9.5 **The morning following his admission Michael refuses his breakfast and the nurse is instructed to ensure that he takes a 30 g carbohydrate drink. Michael should be offered:**

a 100 ml of milk and 2 teaspoonfuls of sugar

b 2 dextrose tablets in 50 ml of water

c 1 tablespoon of glucose in 300 ml of milk

d 200 ml of diluted orange juice

9.6 **Michael's diet is to consist of 180 g of carbohydrate. This, however, only accounts for 40% of his total calorie intake. When protein and fat are added the daily calorie intake would be:**

a 1800 kcal (4.2 mJ)

b 2600 kcal (6.2 mJ)

c 4088 kcal (9.7 mJ)

d 4500 kcal (10.7 mJ)

9.7 **While encouraging Michael to continue giving himself his prescribed insulin injections the nurse should also discuss with him the importance of taking his insulin when he:**

a is under emotional stress

b sustains an injury

c undergoes strenuous activity

d suffers a temporary illness

9.8 **The doctor goes to considerable lengths to develop Michael's understanding of his responsibility regarding the insulin and tells him that the insulin should be:**

a injected into a separate site each day

b preceded by testing a specimen of urine

c taken at the prescribed times

d administered using sterilized needles and syringe

9.9 **A mild ketosis is most likely to be caused by the oxidation of fat in the absence of:**

a amino acids

b electrolytes

c glucose

d lipids

9.10 When Michael is weighed he expresses some astonishment at losing 3 kg of bodyweight in less than a week. This weight loss is most probably due to:

a drinking excessive fluids at the expense of food
b a diet far too low in carbohydrates
c pyrexia and episodes of vomiting
d a constantly raised blood sugar level above 10 mmol per litre

10 Gastroenteritis

PATIENT'S PROFILE

Julie is 12 months old and an only child. Her mother has brought her directly to the accident and emergency department of the hospital and is very anxious that her daughter is so ill. In the last 36 hours Julie has had between 12 and 14 very loose bowel motions, and vomited her last few feeds. The baby looks very dehydrated and her recorded temperature is slightly raised. The doctor decides to admit Julie into hospital with a provisional diagnosis of gastroenteritis and indicates the following regimen:

glucose water only by mouth
cloxacillin (Orbenin) 62.5 mg intramuscularly once then 62.5 mg orally (cloxacillin syrup) every 6 hours
isolation nursing
faecal specimens for culture and sensitivity

10.1 The signs of dehydration that Julie is likely to show may include

a irritability, meningism, and bulging anterior fontanelles
b a dry skin, irritability, diarrhoea and vomiting
c weight loss, dry skin and depressed anterior fontanelles
d moist skin, weight loss, diarrhoea and vomiting

10.2 The nurse is asked to record Julie's temperature every 4 hours. The most appropriate site from which to take the body temperature would be the:

a mouth
b rectum
c axilla
d groin

10.3 The causative organism of Julie's diarrhoea is most likely to be:

a *Escherichia coli*
b *Proteus vulgaris*
c *Candida albicans*
d *Treponema pallidum*

10.4 After settling Julie in her cot in the isolation cubicle, Julie's mother is advised she may visit her daughter:

a only in the afternoon visiting period
b when Julie is taken out of isolation
c by arrangement with the ward sister or charge nurse
d either after 10.00 hours or during the early evening

10.5 The dosage of cloxacillin that Julie has been prescribed will depend on:

a the causative organism of the gastroenteritis
b the severity of the diarrhoea and vomiting
c her weight, age and height
d giving the minimum amount of drug for the maximum effect

10.6 The presentation pack of the cloxacillin is 500 mg in 2 ml. To ensure that Julie receives her prescribed dose, the nurse should draw up in the syringe a drug volume of:

a 0.25 ml
b 0.5 ml
c 1 ml
d 1.5 ml

10.7 During her feeds Julie tends to suckle hungrily. To prevent her from swallowing air the nurse could:

a support Julie's head with the neck fully extended
b ensure that the teat is always full
c give Julie a rest after every 10 ml
d regularly burp Julie during the feed

10.8 In conversation with Julie's mother, the nurse learns that she uses a very unreliable method for sterilizing her baby's feeding utensils. The nurse should advise the mother that, after washing and rinsing, the utensils should be:

a left soaking in boiling water for 20 minutes
b put in a hot oven for 30 minutes
c immersed in a mild disinfectant for 60 minutes
d immersed in a mild antiseptic for 60 minutes

10.9 Twenty-four hours after Julie's admission a second child on the main ward develops diarrhoea which is not related to the illness for which he was originally admitted. The possible cause of cross-infection from Julie to this second child is that:

a Julie's illness is airborne
b the nursing staff are vectors
c food is being shared by the children
d preparation of the milk feeds is unhygienic

10.10 Vomiting is a reflex action coordinated by the:

a cerebellum
b cerebrum
c medulla oblongata
d pons variolii

Surgical Case Histories

11 Pyloric Stenosis

PATIENT'S PROFILE

Timothy was a first child weighing 4.2 kilograms at birth and being physically normal when discharged from the local maternity hospital three weeks ago. Mrs Brasher, Timothy's mother, is now both alarmed and puzzled over her son's tendency to vomit back most of each of his bottle feeds. His persistent crying is agitating her to the point of desperation.

On hearing of Timothy's problem from Mrs Brasher the health visitor arranged for Timothy to have an examination by the doctor at the health centre. Mrs Brasher had to agree with the general practitioner's comments that Timothy had not made any significant weight gain, was moderately dehydrated and slightly pyrexial. When asked to describe the type of vomiting, Mrs Brasher could only express it as being 'very forceful' but 'without any retching'. The vomitus looked like curdled milk and had a rather offensive odour.

On the doctor's recommendation Timothy was admitted to the children's hospital for further tests, to correct his dehydration, and to monitor the pyrexia. The paediatrician, after a thorough examination, prescribed the following regimen for Timothy:

nasogastric aspiration hourly
prepare a test feed
nil orally except for a test feed
intravenous normal saline with 5% Dextrose 100 ml every 2 hours via a scalp infusion
ampicillin (Penbritin) 62.5 mg one injection only intramuscularly
prepare for possible surgery to correct a hypertrophic pyloric stenosis

11.1 **The nurse could help the paediatrician diagnose pyloric stenosis by holding Timothy during:**

- **a** an abdominal X-ray
- **b** intravenous sampling
- **c** gastric aspiration
- **d** a test feed

11.2 On making a definitive diagnosis the paediatrician explained to Mrs Brasher that the name of the operation to correct the stenosis at the pyloric end of the stomach was commonly called:

a Billroth's operation
b Heller's operation
c Ramstedt's operation
d Whipple's operation

11.3 Mrs Brasher was also told that the operation involved making a small incision into Timothy's abdomen over the stomach and:

a removing a small portion of the pyloric end of the stomach to relieve obstruction
b cutting one branch of the vagus nerve supplying the stomach which would relax the pylorus
c incising into but not through the muscle layers of the pyloric end of the stomach
d suturing together the oblique muscle layers of the pylorus

11.4 The prescribed intravenous therapy is intended to correct Timothy's dehydration and:

a his becoming more acidotic
b alkalosis and ketosis
c parenteral drug route
d his episodic vomiting

11.5 To minimize the risk of a localized postoperative complication the one major symptom which must be dealt with in the preoperative phase is:

a vomiting
b dehydration
c toxaemia
d gastritis

11.6 While waiting to accompany Timothy to the operating theatre, Mrs Brasher asks the nurse what the cause of pyloric stenosis was thought to be. The most correct answer to this question is that pyloric stenosis is:

a a congenital defect commonly affecting male infants

b a familial disease equally distributed between male and female children

c a genetically transmitted disorder occurring in large families

d incidental with very little known of its actual cause

11.7 Ampicillin is an antibiotic and has most probably been prescribed:

a as a prophylactic measure

b to treat the gastritis

c to resolve the pyrexia

d to prevent toxaemia

11.8 Two hours after surgery Timothy is prescribed 5 ml of oral glucose saline to be given every hour for the next 3 hours. Glucose saline is normally preferred for the initial postoperative feeding regimen because it:

a is non irritant to the peritoneum

b is readily absorbed by the gastric mucosa

c has a high carbohydrate content

d is readily aspirated in case of vomiting

11.9 Thirty-six hours after surgery the nurse could reassure Mrs Brasher that the operation appears to have been successful because Timothy:

a has had a bowel motion

b is to have intravenous therapy discontinued

c has made some gain in bodyweight

d is feeding contentedly

11.10 On Timothy's discharge from hospital Mrs Brasher should be advised that the immediate care of her son will now be dealt with by the:

a district nurse

b general practitioner

c health visitor

d paediatric liaison officer

12 Partial Gastrectomy

PATIENT'S PROFILE

Mr Swanson is a 32-year-old bachelor and has a 4-year history of chronic dyspepsia which responded to conservative treatment of antacids and a suitable diet. More recently his symptoms of heartburn and dyspepsia have become very troublesome and have not responded to carbenoxolone sodium. Several days ago Mr Swanson was admitted to hospital with a mild degree of haematemesis. After a few days' bedrest his physician requested a barium meal X-ray and referred Mr Swanson for a surgical opinion. The barium meal conclusively showed severe ulceration of the posterior wall of the stomach.

After a careful examination the surgeon advised Mr Swanson that the best course of action to cure his condition would be a partial gastrectomy to which Mr Swanson agreed. The surgeon indicated on Mr Swanson's notes that surgery was listed to take place in 2 days' time. He also requested:

2 units of blood to be grouped and crossmatched
a nasogastric tube to be passed 1 hour before surgery

12.1 **Mr Swanson's gastric ulcer is most likely to be located:**

a on the greater curvature of the stomach
b at the junction of the pylorus and duodenum
c on the lesser curvature of the stomach
d at the junction of the cardia and the oesophagus

12.2 **The day before his operation Mr Swanson was given a detailed account of the events which would precede and follow surgery. The nurse gives this advice knowing that research has quantitatively proven that such advice will:**

a increase the patient's confidence in the surgical team and nursing staff
b help the patient to monitor his own progress
c help the patient put his natural anxieties into true perspective
d reduce the total amount of postoperative analgesia required

12.3 **As part of his prescribed premedication Mr Swanson is to receive atropine 0.6 mg intramuscularly. This drug will:**

a constrict the pupils of the eyes
b decrease the heart rate
c reduce acinar secretions
d induce drowsiness

12.4 **When passing a nasogastric tube the nurse advises Mr Swanson to start swallowing when the tip of the tube is:**

a resting on the upper nasal cavity
b felt to be in the pharynx
c resting in the posterior nasal cavity
d felt to be in the oropharynx

12.5 **Mr Swanson's operation of a simple partial gastrectomy may also be referred to as:**

a Heller's operation
b Billroth's operation
c gastrojejunostomy
d vagotomy and pyloroplasty

12.6 **The nurse is asked to aspirate the stomach contents every hour postoperatively. For the first few hours small amounts of altered blood are aspirated. This is probably due to:**

a internal haemorrhage
b an insecure anastomosis
c over-transfusion of blood
d the surgical procedure

12.7 **On the second postoperative day the surgeon requests that the nasogastric tube be removed. While doing this the nurse pinches the tube along its length to:**

a prevent air entering the stomach
b reduce the risk of nausea and vomiting
c prevent the tube contents entering the larynx
d provide better control over the tube

12.8 Mr Swanson suffered from a 40-minute bout of hiccoughs which was relieved by an injection of chlorpromazine (Largactil). Hiccoughs are due to a spasmodic contraction of the:

a oropharynx
b oesophagus
c diaphragm
d larynx

12.9 As he recovers and takes an increased interest in his diet Mr Swanson should be advised that, while he can eventually enjoy a normal diet, the amount he eats at each meal may be smaller than the average, because of an increased risk of:

a dumping syndrome
b hiatus hernia
c recurring ulceration
d pernicious anaemia

12.10 The cause of gastric ulceration is thought to be:

a excess secretion of hydrochloric acid and reduced secretion of mucus
b excessive nicotine and alcohol indulgence
c increased anxiety and prolonged psychological stress
d irregular dietary habits and incorrect nutritional intake

13 Inguinal Hernia

PATIENT'S PROFILE

Roger Simpkin, now 50 years old, has been a delivery milkman all of his adult working life. In the last few months he has become increasingly aware of an acute dragging pain in the right groin. Whenever he lifts a milk crate or stretches he is constantly reminded of the pain which, so far, has been tolerable.

The company that he works for insists that their employees have an annual medical check after the age of 48 years. It is at such a medical examination that the doctor tells Roger he has a hernia and advises him to visit his own general practitioner.

Roger's doctor agrees with the diagnosis and organizes that Roger's name be placed on the waiting list at the local hospital. He explains to Roger that he has a rupture of the muscle which a small operation will easily correct. In the meantime Roger is strongly advised to avoid heavy lifting, to reduce his weight by at least 17 kilograms and to cut down on his habit of smoking 15 cigarettes per day, which will help to get rid of his early morning cough.

13.1 Mr Simpkin is admitted to hospital for a simple repair of an inguinal hernia. This operation is also known as an:

a herniotomy
b herniorraphy
c hernioplasty
d herniocele

13.2 The underlying cause of Roger's hernia is:

a being overweight by 17 kilograms
b abdominal strain due to coughing
c a congenital defect of the inguinal canal
d abdominal strain due to heavy lifting

13.3 Roger's hernia is described as a rupture of the muscular wall which allows the contents of the abdominal cavity to escape:

a through the femoral ring
b outwards against the umbilicus
c via the linea alba
d towards the scrotal sac

13.4 After a physical examination the surgeon remarks on how difficult it is to 'reduce' the hernia during abdominal palpation. If the hernia is said to be 'irreducible' it is:

a gangrenous
b incarcerated
c obstructed
d oedematous

13.5 During his recovery from the anaesthetic Mr Simpkin suddenly has a respiratory spasm and becomes cyanotic. The nurses' immediate action would be to:

a administer oxygen
b check the radial and carotid pulses
c apply upward pressure to the upper mandible
d adjust Mr Simpkin's position

13.6 A major problem that Mr Simpkin experiences postoperatively is difficulty in micturition. The most effective nursing measure to help him, would be to:

a offer a urinal at frequent intervals
b encourage him to drink clear fluids
c run tap water within his hearing
d stand him at the bedside

13.7 Mr Simpkin develops an irritating cough. The nurse expresses some concern about this because it is most likely to:

a interfere with his routine chest physiotherapy
b cause a scrotal swelling
c increase intra-abdominal pressure
d irritate other ward patients

13.8 A most useful measure to help Mr Simpkin overcome local discomforts from the operation would be:

a an indwelling urinary catheter
b intermittent gastric aspiration
c continuous scrotal support
d a daily evacuant enema

13.9 In the short term the integrity of Roger's surgical incision is threatened by:

a urinary retention
b scrotal swelling
c overweight
d his employment

13.10 **On discharge from hospital the nurse should emphasize to Roger that to avoid recurrence he should:**

a avoid lifting any weight for several months
b take moderate exercise during his convalescence
c maintain his normal weight
d consider taking early retirement

14 Intestinal Obstruction

PATIENT'S PROFILE

Arthur Simpson, now aged 74 and an ex-miner, is admitted as an emergency to the accident and emergency department with severe abdominal distension and a 48-hour history of vomiting copious amounts of faecal smelling fluid.

On examination he is grossly dehydrated, very confused and restless. His blood pressure is recorded as 12/9 kPa (90/60 mmHg) with a radial pulse of 120 beats per minute. The surgeon on call admits him immediately to the emergency surgical ward for preparation for a laparotomy for a suspected intestinal obstruction. While the theatre is being prepared the doctor requests:

intravenous therapy of normal saline 0.9% with Dextrose 5% 500 ml every 4 hours
grouping and crossmatching of 2 units of blood
full blood count, ESR, blood urea and electrolytes
cephaloridine (Ceporin) 500 mg intramuscular injection every 6 hours
preparation for abdominal surgery

14.1 **The prescribed intravenous fluids could be described as being:**

a hypertonic
b isotopic
c hypotonic
d isotonic

14.2 **Mr Simpson is able to pass a small amount of urine for routine testing and the nurse observes that the volume is not only minute but is also very concentrated. This is because Mr Simpson has:**

a glycosuria
b hypoproteinaemia
c urinary retention
d hypovolaemia

14.3 **The operating theatre staff telephone the ward to advise they will be ready for Mr Simpson in 30 minutes. The most urgent task for the nurse to complete is:**

a to obtain Mr Simpson's written consent to surgery
b to ensure that a unit of blood is available
c to give Mr Simpson a bedbath
d to give Mr Simpson his premedication

14.4 **On his return to the recovery room the nurse is told that Mr Simpson has a temporary colostomy, a midline abdominal incision with stab drain, urinary drainage and a blood transfusion in progress. Which of the following requires greatest care when transferring Mr Simpson from stretcher trolley to bed:**

a the patency of the transfusion
b security of the wound dressing
c activity of the colostomy
d correct positioning of the urinary drainage

14.5 **Mr Simpson is prescribed 1 g of potassium chloride which is to be added to every second unit of infusion fluid, i.e., 1 g in every 1000 ml. This particular drug would specifically help in:**

a promoting urinary excretion
b preventing cardiac arrhythmia
c relaxing involuntary muscle
d encouraging colostomy activity

14.6 Mr Simpson is told by the surgeon that his colostomy is only temporary. He asks the nurse what specifically is meant by temporary. The best answer the nurse could offer to Mr Simpson would be:

a not more than six months to allow the bowel to heal
b until the cause of the bowel obstruction has been diagnosed
c until he has a second elective operation
d until the colostomy is acting normally and regularly

14.7 On the first postoperative day the colostomy appliance should be:

a changed each time the colostomy is active
b pinholed on its upper edge
c securely sealed to the skin at every edge
d changed every 4 hours

14.8 When cleaning the colostomy stoma one important checking procedure the nurse must make is to check the:

a sensitivity of the membrane of the stoma
b integrity of the lumen of the stoma
c integrity of the surrounding skin
d wound drainage is intact

14.9 On the first postoperative day the surgeon requests the nurse carries out a colostomy irrigation. This procedure would help to:

a reduce the oedema of the stoma
b reduce the offensive odour
c promote formed faeces
d stimulate regular evacuation

14.10 To ensure that Mr Simpson received the correct blood group, the one test that would have ensured compatibility between his blood and the donor's blood is to match his:

a antigens with the donor's antibodies
b serum with the donor's erythrocytes
c erythrocytes with the donor's antigens
d agglutinogens with the donor's antigens

15 Ileostomy

PATIENT'S PROFILE

Mr Colin Baker, a 25-year-old bachelor, has had an inflammatory disease of the large colon for over 3 years (ulcerative colitis). For the past 2 years the colitis was kept in remission with the prescribed regimen of steroid therapy and diet. During the last 12 months, however, Colin has had two relapses suffering from frequent loose bowel motions and a marked loss of weight. Typically the bowel motions have been very fluid in nature containing mucus and fresh blood.

His own physician was of the opinion that any altered steroid therapy would no longer remain a satisfactory method of conservative treatment and asked the hospital consultant to consider if surgery would be more appropriate for Colin. The surgeon, after assessing the medical background and evaluating the results of a barium enema and a rectal mucosal biopsy, agreed that Colin should be persuaded to have a total colectomy and a permanent ileostomy. After lengthy discussions, Colin agreed to the operation and was admitted as a waiting list patient three days prior to his planned operation.

15.1 **Colin's 'informed consent' to the operation implies the principle of obtaining his signature on the consent form after the:**

- **a** senior nurse gives a detailed account of preoperative and postoperative care and has witnessed the signing of the consent form
- **b** surgeon has explained the implications of the proposed surgery and has witnessed the signing of the consent form
- **c** anaesthetist has outlined the risks and problems associated with an ileostomy
- **d** consultant has given Colin and his family a detailed account of all the surgical implications

15.2 In the first few days of preparing Colin for his operation, the nurse should be able to guide and inform him about the most appropriate diet. This is most likely to be:

a high protein and high residue
b low protein and low residue
c low protein, low residue and fat-free
d high protein and low residue

15.3 Colin's bowel preparation for the colectomy is most likely to be a:

a rectal washout twice daily for 2 days
b enema saponis each evening for 3 nights
c prednisolone (Predsol) retention enema each evening for 3 nights
d prescribed oral sulphamethizole (Urolucosil) drugs

15.4 Following a total colectomy Colin will not be able to synthesize certain vitamins. These vitamins are:

a A and D
b C and B
c B and K
d C and D

15.5 Within 24 hours of Colin's surgery the nurse could expect that the stoma will:

a expel digested food
b expel a considerable amount of flatus
c expel digestive enzymes
d remain quiescent

15.6 Once the stoma is active the discharge could be expected to excoriate the skin surrounding the stoma. Such excoriation would most likely to be caused by:

a pancreozymin and cholecystokinin
b amylase and lipase
c hydrochloric acid and protease
d cholesterol and mucin

15.7 **During the second postoperative day Colin's stoma is discharging a very large volume of ileal fluid. This may lead to:**

a liver failure
b iron-deficiency anaemia
c negative nitrogen balance
d metabolic acidosis

15.8 **Colin has until now been friendly, courteous and cooperative with the nursing staff. On the second and third postoperative days he has become antagonistic and had several angry outbursts at his nurses. These angry outbursts could be considered as:**

a a natural response to elective major surgery
b a defence mechanism to a damaged libido
c a coping mechanism to altered body image
d evidence of a psychiatrically disturbed patient

15.9 **On the third postoperative day the surgeon prescribes vitamins B and C to supplement Colin's very light diet. The nurse can assume these vitamins will**

a prevent anaemia from occurring
b increase plasma protein viscosity
c promote healing of the wound
d prevent skin excoriation at the stoma site

15.10 **During a discussion with Colin about his stoma appliance, the nurse should place the greatest emphasis upon the:**

a fact that ileal fluid can be regulated to discharge once per day
b need to irrigate the stoma at frequent intervals
c need to apply karaya gum to protect the skin surrounding the stoma
d need to always have spare ileostomy applicances available

16 Ventricular Septal Defect

PATIENT'S PROFILE

Steven, now aged 4 years, has had a ventricular septal defect since he was born. It was first diagnosed at 8 weeks old when he was found during a routine examination to have a heart murmur. In the intervening years he has enjoyed normal development being physically asymptomatic. Both his parents are teachers and are very sensible and reliable about following the advice given by the consultant in charge of Steven's health.

When he was 3 years old Steven had a cardiac catheterization which clearly demonstrated the small defect in the septum between the ventricles of the heart. A chest X-ray also showed the heart to be very enlarged. The cardiologist recommended corrective surgery once Steven had completed his initial immunization programme and had had a dental check.

On admission to the ward Steven and his parents were shown to a single-bedded room and were allowed time to settle in and become acquainted with Steven's new environment. It was explained to Steven's parents that their son could play with the other children in the main ward and these first few days in hospital would be used to complete essential investigations before his operation which was planned for two days later. Steven's mother asked for and was given permission to visit at any time, including sleeping overnight on the day of the operation.

Steven was a shy boy but cooperated when the nurse undressed him for his first test which was an electrocardiogram, then later he had an echogram. The phlebotomist collected blood specimens for blood-grouping and crossmatching and a full blood count which was not well tolerated by Steven who had to be gently restrained by the nurses during the procedure.

After a very careful physical examination the surgeon spent a long time detailing the operation to Steven's parents. He described the need for firstly giving premedication, the use of the cardiopulmonary bypass machine, and how they would repair the defect with a material known as filamentous dacron. During the operation icepacks would be used to keep the local temperature below normal body temperature, and if all went well the total operation time would be about 2 hours. After the operation Steven would be cared for in the coronary care unit for 2 days because he would have a tube coming from his chest wall, a tube from his bladder, another into his stomach which the nurses would aspirate to keep the stomach empty and another tube into his veins into which fluid would be given. The parents gave their written consent to closure of ventricular septal defect realizing it was a major operation.

16.1 Steven was diagnosed as having a cardiac defect on the basis of a 'cardiac murmur'. This term implies that there was incomplete:

a emptying of the right auricle
b closing of the aortic valve
c emptying of the ventricles
d closing of the mitral valve

16.2 The principal purpose of a dental check would be to:

a eradicate the presence of *Streptococcus viridans*
b ensure normal orthodontic development
c treat existing dental caries
d identify loose teeth

16.3 Droperidol (Droleptan) was administered as the prescribed premedication. This drug would effectively induce:

a dissociative anaesthesia
b euphoria and sedation
c neuroleptoanalgesia
d anxiolytic sedation

16.4 During surgery the sequence of surgical incisions to reach the defect would be:

a median sternotomy, pericardiotomy, right ventriculotomy
b right ventriculotomy, median sternotomy, pericardiotomy
c pericardiotomy, right ventriculotomy, median sternotomy
d right ventriculotomy, pericardiotomy, median sternotomy

16.5 When the cardiopulmonary bypass machine was used, Steven's venous blood was taken to the machine via two venous cannulae and returned to his body via one arterial cannula. The blood vessels most likely to be cannulated are the:

a inferior and superior vena cavae and aorta
b carotid and brachial arteries and inferior vena cava
c pulmonary artery, inferior and superior vena cavae
d carotid artery, inferior and superior vena cavae

16.6 **The septal defect was repaired over a total period of 48 minutes at a local temperature of 25°C. The blood vessel which is clamped off during this time is the:**

a right coronary artery
b pulmonary vein
c aorta
d left coronary artery

16.7 **Prior to closing the pericardium Steven's heart went into ventricular tachycardia. This is normally corrected by:**

a cardiac massage
b defibrillation
c intravenous adrenaline
d intravenous digoxin

16.8 **At the conclusion of surgery, the cardiopulmonary machine was switched off, the natural circulation restored and the ice packs removed. The main complication which might occur at this time is:**

a coronary thrombosis
b pericardial rupture
c sinus arrhythmia
d pulmonary collapse

16.9 **For the first 24 hours of postoperative care Steven had his stomach emptied via nasogastric aspiration because it:**

a reduces the body's metabolic needs
b minimizes existing paralytic ileus
c minimizes gastric motility
d reduces intra-abdominal pressure

16.10 **Steven's urinary output was carefully monitored for 48 hours. The reason for this is that the kidneys receive 25% of the cardiac output. Given that Steven has a circulatory volume of 3 litres, the volume received by the kidneys is:**

a 550 ml
d 650 ml
c 750 ml
d 850 ml

17 Splenectomy

PATIENT'S PROFILE

Joe, at 16, was given the opportunity to play for the local football club in the junior's reserve team and succeeded in being offered an apprenticeship. A few weeks after joining the club he was learning tackling techniques when he was inadvertently but forcefully kicked in the upper abdomen. Apart from being winded and bruised he temporarily recovered and continued to practice. A few hours later he complained to the manager that he felt giddy, very cold and had worsening abdominal pain. Without further ado the manager brought Joe to the accident and emergency department where the medical officer referred Joe to the surgeon on call.

An examination showed that Joe had a low body temperature and his blood pressure and pulse were within normal limits. His respirations were shallow and painful but a plain chest and abdominal X-ray did not reveal any abnormalities. Joe's appearance was one of a person in shock and the surgeon admitted Joe with a suspected splenic injury and advised the following regimen:

- bedrest
- hourly observations of pulse, blood pressure and abdominal girth
- group and crossmatch 2 units of AB blood rhesus-positive
- haematocrit
- nil by mouth
- ampicillin (Penbritin) 250 mg intramuscularly every 4 hours for 5 days

17.1 At the time of his admission the type of shock from which Joe was suffering could be described as being:

a traumatic, neurogenic and cardiogenic
b vasomotor, primary and splenic
c hypotensive, haemorrhagic and neurogenic
d traumatic, psychogenic and hypotensive

17.2 Two hours after Joe was admitted the surgeon carried out a second examination and advised the nurse that he suspected a splenic haematoma. The nurse should know that the pain from such an injury is located in the left upper abdomen and radiates to the:

- a right upper abdominal region
- b subscapular region
- c whole abdominal musculature
- d lower thoracic cavity and epigastrium

17.3 The haematocrit is an investigation which determines the:

- a volume percentage of erythrocytes in whole blood
- b erythrocyte percentage in a given volume of plasma
- c plasma viscosity and differential count
- d volume percentage of plasma following haemorrhage

17.4 A splenic haematoma may rupture within 72 hours of its occurrence. The signs that require an immediate surgical opinion are:

- a bleeding into the peritoneal cavity
- b tachycardia and marked hypotension
- c an abnormal haematocrit
- d pain in the left upper abdominal quadrant

17.5 Following surgery Joe was transferred with 2 units of blood. The observations which indicate an allergic response include:

- a backache, hypotension, breathlessness, oliguria
- b haematuria, shock, vomiting, venospasm
- c oliguria, hypertension, thrombophlebitis, backache
- d nausea, pruritis, skin rash, pyrexia

17.6 To compensate for the loss of the spleen the body responds by:

- a increasing the production of leucocytes
- b becoming increasingly prone to infection
- c having a persistently low blood pressure
- d displacing related abdominal structures

17.7 Seven days after surgery the sutures of Joe's wound were removed. Before being removed the sutures are cut below the knot before being pulled free from the skin. This technique is principally used to avoid:

- a causing further trauma to the wound
- b contamination of the incision line
- c disrupting the healing process
- d causing a haematoma below the incision line

17.8 The total amount of ampicillin which Joe will receive amounts to:

- a 7.5 g and the drug is the same as benzylpenicillin
- b 15 g and the drug is penicillinase resistant
- c 7.5 g and a wide ranging bactericide
- d 15 g and the drug causes a 10% risk of allergic response

17.9 Immediately prior to his discharge Joe should be advised to:

- a ensure that he completes his course of antibiotics
- b take precautions against persistent hypotension
- c consider alternative employment
- d consult his physiotherapist

17.10 The principal function of the spleen is the:

- a production of erythrocytes
- b contribution to body immunity
- c reservoir for venous blood
- d destruction of harmful bacteria

18 Hydrocephalus

PATIENT'S PROFILE

Cheryl, now aged 20 weeks, is to be admitted to hospital with a diagnosis of hydrocephalus and is to have an operation to insert a Spitz–Holter valve which will drain excess cerebrospinal fluid from the brain to reduce increasing intracranial pressure.

Born prematurely, and a twin, Cheryl was for the first 7 weeks of her life nursed in the intensive baby care unit. There she received assisted ventilation and parental feeding until she could breathe independently and suckle effectively. After her discharge from hospital she seemed to make reasonable progress until her 16th week when she suffered from pyrexial bouts accompanied by convulsions. She was given an immediate assessment in the outpatients paediatric clinic where it was noted her cranial circumference was disproportionate to the facial bones and the cranial sutures and fontanelles were widely distended. At this point surgery could not be offered because Cheryl was failing to thrive and was severely underweight.

At 20 weeks old Cheryl reached the required weight of 4 kg, but by this time had developed a convergent squint and had the typical 'setting-sun sign' of hydrocephalic children.

Mrs Rowan, Cheryl's mother, decided to accept hospital residency while her daughter was in hospital and would give Cheryl all the basic infant care which she would require. She had accepted her daughter's handicap with great equanimity and had been well-supported throughout the past 20 weeks by the medical and nursing members of the caring team.

18.1 **Cheryl was admitted into an isolation cubicle although she had no apparent infection. This precaution is taken because:**

- **a** it is recommended by the Department of Health and Social Security
- **b** infection is a high risk with this type of operation
- **c** hydrocephalic children can upset normal children and their parents
- **d** Cheryl has an underdeveloped immune system

18.2 **The first signs of hydrocephalus are usually accepted as being:**

- **a** convergent squint
- **b** convulsions and pyrexia
- **c** disproportionate cranial circumference
- **d** 'setting-sun sign' of the pupils of the eye

18.3 Hydrocephalus is most commonly defined as being due to an:

a overall increase in the cranial diameter
b increased intracranial pressure and excessive cerebrospinal fluid
c obstruction in the flow of cerebrospinal fluid
d obstruction at the base of the fourth ventricle

18.4 A Spitz–Holter valve normally drains cerebrospinal fluid from the:

a lateral ventricles into the venous system
b subarachnoid space into the lateral ventricles
c fourth ventricle into the arterial system
d subarachnoid space into the venous system

18.5 Cheryl suffered from a convergent squint. This is due to pressure on the:

a trigeminal nerve
b third cranial nerve
c sixth cranial nerve
d twelfth cranial nerve

18.6 Cheryl's general anaesthetic consisted of halothane (Fluothane) 2%. The principal advantage of this type of anaesthetic gas is that it has a:

a rapid induction with minimal postoperative emesis and rapid recovery of cough reflex
b slow induction and prolonged postoperative analgesic effect on recovery
c rapid hypotensive action with rapid induction and a slow recovery time
d slow induction, minimal postoperative nausea and a rapid recovery time

18.7 Following recovery from surgery Cheryl was given paracetamol syrup to control her agitation and restlessness. This drug counters the discomforts of:

a pain, inflammation and pyrexia
b vomiting, pyrexia and inflammation
c pain, nausea and diarrhoea
d hiccoughs, pain and nausea

18.8 **Postoperative observations would also include noting if the Spitz–Holter valve was:**
- a a source of local infection
- b becoming blocked
- c causing cardiac irritation
- d interfering with swallowing and feeding

18.9 **The tubing attached to the Spitz–Holter valve would usually drain the excess cerebrospinal fluid into the:**
- a left atrium
- b carotid artery
- c internal jugular vein
- d right atrium

18.10 **Mrs Rowan asked the nurse if this type of surgery was a 'once and for all' technique. The most correct answer would be to say that:**
- a apart from regular checks on growth and development no further surgery is usually carried out
- b if there was a spontaneous recovery in the normal flow of cerebrospinal fluid the valve could then be removed
- c at regular intervals the valve and tubing would require replacing
- d at regular intervals the tubing attached to the valve would be lengthened

19 Appendicitis

PATIENT'S PROFILE

Simon, aged 4, has been brought to the accident and emergency department by his mother who is very anxious about her son's rather sudden illness. In the last four hours Simon has refused food and drink, is slightly pyrexial, has vomited twice and become rather fretful and listless.

After an examination the casualty officer decides to admit Simon for observation with a provisional diagnosis of appendicitis. He asks for routine observations and prescribes one dose of ampicillin (Penbritin) 125 mg by intramuscular injection and then 62.5 mg per ml oral ampicillin for ten doses. He also asks that the surgical registrar be contacted to urgently examine Simon in more detail if his condition appears to become worse.

19.1 The abdominal pain initially and classically associated with appendicitis occurs in the:

a epigastrium and right iliac fossa
b right hypochondrium and right iliac fossa
c right iliac fossa
d umbilical region and right iliac fossa

19.2 The appendix is attached to the:

a ileum
b ileocaecal valve
c caecum
d colon

19.3 Appendicitis is more serious in Simon's case because in children of his age the:

a appendix is more difficult to mobilize and remove by surgery
b local inflammation and infection may disseminate
c lymphoid tissue of the appendix is not fully developed
d appendix is inadequately protected by the greater omentum

19.4 From the prescribed ampicillin it can be calculated that Simon will receive a total amount of:

a 0.570 g
b 0.750 g
c 5.750 g
d 7.500 g

19.5 The most accurate description of appendicitis is that it is an inflammation:

a resulting from obstruction of the lumen of the appendix
b arising spontaneously within the appendix
c caused by pathogenic bacteria in the caecum
d arising from lymphoid tissue hyperplasia

19.6 **The nurse would be quite clear in her mind of the need to summon the registrar quickly if Simon's temperature:**

a rose, the pulse became more rapid and he had less abdominal pain

b fell, the pulse became more rapid and the abdominal pain increased

c rose and the pulse remained the same with the abdominal pain becoming dull

d fell, the pulse became more rapid and Simon complained of colic-type pain

19.7 **The registrar decided that Simon required an emergency appendicectomy. The nurse advised Simon's mother that if at all possible she should try to be with Simon on his recovery from anaesthesia. This is because:**

a a familiar face is the best reassurance for a child in hospital

b it reinforces the mother–child bond relationship

c it will reduce Simon's anxiety when awakening in a strange environment

d it continues the existing mother–child relationship

19.8 **Following surgery the instruction is given 'nil by mouth' until bowel sounds are heard. Such an instruction implies that Simon may start oral fluids when:**

a he has had a bowel motion

b he has passed flatus

c peristaltic waves can be seen

d peristalsis is detected by stethoscope

19.9 **The surgeon used a grid-iron incision to open Simon's abdomen. This incision is usually located over the:**

a para-umbilical region

b hypochondrium

c hypogastrium

d right iliac region

19.10 **Simon's wound healed without complication by:**

a first intention

b granulation

c primary suture

d second intention

20 Cholecystectomy

PATIENT'S PROFILE

Mrs Janet Colby is a 35-year-old housewife who is normally a jolly, inquisitive person. She prides herself in keeping a good home and in her well-fed husband and four children. In the last few months Janet has been aware of abdominal discomfort especially in the right upper abdomen. She has noticed increasingly that not only is the pain getting worse but she has bouts of vomiting and feels sick most of the time. Her own doctor suspects she has biliary disease and requests a hospital outpatients appointment for her.

A straight abdominal X-ray shows suspicious stones in the gallbladder and her serum bilirubin is raised. The consultant advises her to take a fat-free diet until she can be admitted to hospital for further investigations. On her admission from the waiting list the only surgical instruction is that she is for a cholecystogram the following morning with a view to cholecystectomy in two days' time.

20.1 The nurse observes that Janet's skin is slightly tinged with a yellow colour. This may suggest that the stones are situated in the:

a cystic duct
b common bile duct
c hepatic duct
d gallbladder

20.2 On enquiry Janet admits that she does have pruritis. This irritation may be relieved with the application of:

a calomel solution
b calamine lotion
c camphor oil
d cetrimide solution

20.3 **Janet was fasted overnight in preparation for her cholecystogram. During the X-ray she will be offered either richly buttered toast or a similar fatty type of meal. The reason for this is that the meal will:**

a stimulate the gallbladder to contract
b help to concentrate the radiopaque dye in the gallbladder
c stimulate the liver to secrete bile during the X-ray
d absorb and help to excrete the dye from the body after the X-ray

20.4 **The cholecystogram confirms the presence of stones in the biliary tract and gallbladder and Janet's operation is confirmed to take place. The surgeon prescribes vitamin K injections preoperatively and postoperatively. The most likely reason for such injections is that the vitamin K will:**

a decrease the serum bilirubin level
b reduce the risk of bleeding
c reduce the risk of thrombosis
d decrease the platelet count

20.5 **The nurse explains to Janet that a cholecystectomy is the removal of the gallbladder which, when healthy, has the normal function of:**

a producing bile
b concentrating bile
c absorbing bile
d secreting bile

20.6 **Janet is puzzled as to why she must have vitamin K by injection and not with her food. The nurse could explain that vitamin K can only be absorbed by the gut in the presence of:**

a serum bilirubin
b cholecystokinin
c bile salts
d bile pigments

20.7 Janet makes a reasonable recovery from her surgery but is puzzled and uncomfortable by the presence of the T tube secured by suture into her wound. The nurse should be able to explain that the primary purpose of this tube is that it:

a will eventually be required to do a postoperative cholangiogram
b measures the volume of bile being secreted from the wound
c acts as a bypass in the very oedematous bile duct
d acts as a safety valve in case of postoperative biliary obstruction

20.8 Nursing measures in the first few postoperative days include those which will prevent the common complications of:

a thrombophlebitis and hypotension
b abdominal distension and chest infection
c renal failure and diarrhoea
d burst abdomen and deep vein thrombosis

20.9 The surgeon requests that a postoperative cholangiogram is done before the T tube is removed. This procedure is normally done to establish whether the:

a T tube is patent
b operative site has healed
c common bile duct is patent
d serum bilirubin is normal

20.10 Before her discharge from hospital Janet is advised to take things gently for the next 4 weeks and to encourage her family to do most of the household chores. This advice is given to avoid the possibility of:

a chest infection
b rupture of wound
c incisional hernia
d wound infection

Orthopaedic Case Histories

21 Fracture of the Radius and Ulna

PATIENT'S PROFILE

On her 11th birthday Mandy was given a bicycle as a present from her parents. For the first few weeks Mandy's parents were quite strict about where she could practice cycling, until she completed a cycling proficiency course organized by the local constabulary. On her first solo outing Mandy tried to avoid a collision with another cyclist. She had the presence of mind to guide the front wheel of her bicycle towards the pavement but in doing this lost her balance, falling onto her left side and trapping her arm under her bodyweight. The rear wheel and mudguard of the bicycle also caused minor abrasions of her left knee and calf muscles.

On arrival at the accident and emergency department Mandy could not remember the accident nor could she give details of her name or where she lived. Her left wrist was flaccidly flexed and when the doctor tried to examine Mandy's arm she cried out in pain. After an X-ray the doctor confirmed a simple fracture of the left radius and ulna, which would require to be immobilized in a plaster cast. He also requested that Mandy be admitted for 24 hours and before being admitted to the ward should be given:

penicillin 2 000 000 units intramuscularly
tetanus toxoid
wound toilet to her left leg

In the meantime the sister informed the police that an unidentified child had been admitted to hospital following a minor road traffic accident.

21.1 A flaccidly flexed wrist also known as a 'dinner fork deformity' is usually indicative of:

a Colles' fracture
b Bennett's fracture
c Pott's fracture
d Smith's fracture

21.2 **When undressing Mandy for her examination the nurse should remove her clothing by starting to undress her:**

a from her right side

b from her left side

c by cutting along the seams of her clothing

d by taking her clothing over her head

21.3 **Before Mandy arrives on the ward she has a plaster cast applied to her arm from elbow to wrist. The ward nurse will ensure that the plaster dries satisfactorily by:**

a testing the cast with the palmar surface of the hand

b arranging a suitable airflow with a multidirectional fan

c checking the radial pulse at frequent intervals

d correct positioning of the limb on a waterproof firm pillow

21.4 **Other than observing the plaster of Paris the nurse is requested to make routine observations. Which one of the following would require immediate medical intervention:**

a a low blood pressure

b an absent radial pulse of the left arm

c unequal and dilated pupils

d return of Mandy's memory

21.5 **Mandy complains of an irritating itch of her skin beneath the plaster cast. The nurse should consider that:**

a a window should be cut into the plaster over the area of itching

b the plaster needs to be bivalved

c Mandy should move and exercise her fingers at frequent intervals

d a pressure sore might be developing

21.6 **On checking Mandy's pupils the nurse is observing for a normal reaction to light. The expected normal reaction is:**

a the pupils remain the same size

b the pupils dilate equally and then constrict

c the pupils constrict equally and then dilate

d both pupils remain dilated after being stimulated by light

21.7 The radius and ulna are examples of:

a irregular bones
b flat bones
c long bones
d short bones

21.8 When Mandy's mother eventually arrives at the hospital after being notified by the police of her daughter's accident, the first emotional reaction which the nurse could expect from the mother is:

a depression
b anger
c guilt
d hysteria

21.9 Before Mandy is discharged home the most important instruction which should be given to her mother is to:

a protect the plaster cast with polythene sheeting during bath-time to prevent it from becoming wet
b encourage Mandy to extend and flex the fingers of the affected arm at regular intervals
c keep the affected arm and plaster cast well supported in a sling for at least 7 days
d rest the arm in a sling until the plaster cast is dry

21.10 The main cause of accidents to 11-year-old children occur with the highest incidence:

a in the home
b on main roads
c in school playgrounds
d in rivers and main waterways

22 Rheumatoid Arthritis

PATIENT'S PROFILE

Mrs Butler, aged 32, has been admitted to the medical ward with a diagnosis of acute rheumatoid arthritis. At the time of admission she complains of severe pain and limited movement of the affected joints. She has a history of rheumatoid arthritis but this has been in remission for some time. The consultant is admitting her for further investigations, treatment, and to give Mr Butler some respite from caring for his wife which he has been doing for the past 3 weeks. The medical notes indicate:

ESR
Rheumatoid Factor Test
acetylsalicylate acid 300–600 mg as required
prednisolone on a sliding scale:
- 25 mg twice daily for 10 days
- 25 mg once daily for 7 days
- 15 mg once daily for 3 days
- maintenance dose to be decided

22.1 During the acute phase of rheumatoid arthritis it is vital that Mrs Butler has:

a armchair rest during the daytime with active physiotherapy to the affected joints
b bedrest with passive physiotherapy to the unaffected joints
c complete bedrest with the affected joints resting in their optimal position
d wheelchair dependency during the day with heat therapy to the affected joints

22.2 Mrs Butler's joint pains and immobility are described as being classical. This means that the affected joints are:

a moderately painful in the morning and worsening as the day progresses
b tolerable at all times so long as the joints are at rest
c tolerable in the morning but increasingly painful at night
d very bad in the morning with some improvement as the day progresses

22.3 In conversation with Mrs Butler the nurse notices that she keeps referring to her illness as osteoarthritis. The nurse could help Mrs Butler by explaining that rheumatoid arthritis is:

a an inflammation of the weight-bearing joints and is asymmetrical in pattern
b affects only the small joints and is symmetrical in pattern
c is a progressive infective inflammation of the small joints
d is also known as polyarthritis, i.e., inflammation of many joints

22.4 Acetylsalicylate acid would help Mrs Butler because this drug is an:

a autoimmune suppressive agent
b analgesic and antipyretic
c antiallergen
d antirheumatoid agent

22.5 If the rheumatoid factor is present in Mrs Butler's blood sample this might indicate that:

a a raised factor level shows that other tissues are involved
b a very low reading confirms the diagnosis of rheumatoid arthritis
c its presence establishes a unique diagnosis of rheumatoid arthritis
d its presence shows that other diseases may coexist with rheumatoid arthritis

22.6 In Mrs Butler's case the erythrocyte sedimentation rate is likely to be:

a 3–5 mm per hour
b 4–7 mm per hour
c 7–12 mm per hour
d 10–15 mm per hour

22.7 If the ESR is raised this would occur because the:

a coagulation factors have increased in their viscosity
b erythrocyte count is raised
c erythrocytes have increased in their viscosity
d leucocyte count is raised

22.8 The prednisolone administered to Mrs Butler may help because this drug is:

a antiallergen and an anti-inflammatory agent
b antibiotic and antispasmodic
c antipyretic and analgesic
d an antirheumatoid factor

22.9 Assuming that Mrs Butler received all the doses of the prescribed prednisolone (sliding scale) what is the total amount of drug taken:

a 0.720 g
b 1.720 g
c 7.220 g
d 72.20 g

22.10 On discharge Mrs Butler is given one week's supply of prednisolone, and advised to contact her own general practitioner for a further prescription which will last for 3 months. Mrs Butler asks whether she will have to pay the full cost of the prescription. The nurse could correctly answer that:

a the patient only has to pay the nominal fee not the full charge
b since the patient is permanently disabled there is no charge at all
c the patient must pay the full current prescription charges
d the prescription must be paid for but in Mrs Butler's case the charges are much reduced

23 Below Knee Amputation

PATIENT'S PROFILE

Roger Atkins, aged 49, a private building contractor has been troubled over the last 18 months with pain in the right leg muscle when walking any distance. He smokes about 30 cigarettes a day but only has an occassional drink, preferably whisky, and is slightly overweight.

On a visit to his general practitioner he agreed that the pain tended to disappear after a rest. The doctor also noted a distinct difference in the temperature between the feet, the right being colder than the left, and also commented upon a demarcation line across the right foot. He advised Roger that he suspected peripheral arterial disease but would refer him for further tests at the hospital.

Following a right femoral arteriogram and a physical tolerance test the surgeon advised Roger that the blood supply to his right foot was inadequate and the only treatment he could offer was a below knee amputation to avoid the possible complication of gangrene.

After a great deal of discussion with his wife about the future outlook Roger gave his consent to the operation. He was then given detailed advice about his personal preparation for this major operation and the preliminary details about the proposed artificial limb. On admission to the ward two weeks later the surgeon requested:

grouping and crossmatching of 4 units of blood
measurement of the right leg for the artificial limb
electrocardiogram
electrolyte and blood urea levels

23.1 The type of pain and history that Roger complains of is typical of:

a Homans' sign
b Raynaud's disease
c Buerger's disease
d varicose veins

23.2 Mr Atkins would be advised in the preoperative stage to:

a avoid alcohol and smoking
b reduce his weight
c give up his cigarettes
d wear elasticated hosiery when walking

23.3 During the preoperative phase the nurse should place the greatest emphasis on the discomfort which will arise from:

a the blood transfusion
b toileting difficulties
c phantom pain
d stump bandaging

23.4 **Twenty-four hours after surgery ambulation will be encouraged to prevent the loss of:**
a muscle tone
b muscle mass
c body coordination
d body image

23.5 **Following amputation the immediate danger to Mr Atkins' recovery would be:**
a flexion deformity
b infection
c secondary haemorrhage
d shock

23.6 **The nurse reported severe blood staining of the stump bandaging 6 hours after surgery. Such haemorrhage is described as:**
a accidental
b primary
c reactionary
d secondary

23.7 **Forty-eight hours after surgery Mr Atkins was introduced to the use of crutches. When learning to use these he should be advised to take the weight of his body from the:**
a shoulders
b axilla
c wrists
d hands

23.8 **To prevent flexion deformity of the stump the nurse would:**
a advise Mr Atkins to contract the knee joint at frequent intervals
b supply firm conical shaped bandaging to the stump
c maintain knee extension by the use of sandbags
d position Roger in the prone position twice daily for 20 minutes

23.9 Ten days after surgery Roger is fitted with a temporary prosthetic limb. The most useful advice the nurse could give at this stage of recovery would be for Roger to:

a apply the bandage before fitting the stump into the cup of the prosthesis

b keep the stump thoroughly clean and dry at all times

c continue using the crutches until more confident with this prosthesis

d graduate the time intervals when wearing the prosthesis until his balance is perfect

23.10 Prior to his transfer to a remedial centre Mr Atkins asks who could advise him on his future employment potential in the building industry. Such a person is the:

a physiotherapist

b medical social worker

c district rehabilitation officer

d consultant orthopaedic surgeon

24 Midshaft Femur Fracture

PATIENT'S PROFILE

Jonathan is a 17-year-old apprentice mechanic who, while travelling to work, was involved in a road traffic accident. Apparently a car travelling at some speed braked suddenly to give way to oncoming traffic and Jonathan rammed into the back of the now stationary car. Jonathan was thrown forwards over the moped handlebars, he fell sideways and his moped fell on top of him.

In the accident and emergency department the examination by X-ray shows an oblique fracture of the midshaft of his right femur, a more detailed examination reveals no other injury. Relieved of his pain by diamorphine 10 mg Jonathan was taken immediately to theatre for an open reduction of the fracture under general anaesthetic and the injured limb was then secured by fixed traction to a Thomas splint.

24.1 At ward report the sister asks a nurse to define what is meant by the term 'fracture reduction'. This is best defined as:

a the removal of bone fragments from the fractured site
b the removal of damaged periosteum from the fractured bone
c surgical manipulation of the affected bones to align the fractured ends
d manual manipulation of the fractured bone to align the broken ends

24.2 Jonathan has fixed traction. To which of the following should the nurse give priority:

a maintaining his morale during the prolonged healing and required bedrest
b preventing infection to which he might be prone
c maintaining his comfort by daily attention to his hygienic needs
d checking and if necessary repadding the ring of the Thomas splint

24.3 Pressure from the fixed traction will be greatest at the:

a ischial tuberosity
b sacral area
c groin
d internal malleolus

24.4 The nurse observes that the foot of Jonathan's bed has been elevated and that the end of the splint has been secured to the bedrail. It would be correct to assume that this:

a will relieve pressure on the groin
b increases countertraction
c maintains abduction of the right leg
d permits flexion of the right knee

24.5 Jonathan's traction is checked every day. Which alteration would require the doctor's permission if the nurse felt it required adjusting:

a abduction of the right leg
b medial rotation of the right leg
c reapplying supporting slings and padding
d replacing traction cord

24.6 Jonathan, being mechanically minded, asks the nurse what the advantage is of his type of traction as opposed to sliding (balance) traction:

a if necessary he could be easily moved from his bed
b it permits the fractured bone to heal at a more rapid rate
c there is less need for padding or joint support
d the pressure at the groin is much less

24.7 On checking the traction cord the nurse observes that to maintain its tension it requires to be adjusted. The best method of correcting the tension would be to:

a increase the weight at the end of the splint
b twist the incorporated windlass
c increase the weight at the upper end of the splint
d increase the elevation at the foot of the bed

24.8 The slings supporting Jonathan's right leg are secured to the lateral aspect of the splint by kilt pins (or similar device). The reason for this is that the:

a kilt pins require daily adjustment
b pins will not rub against the medial aspect of the left leg
c pins exert tension upwards thereby supporting the fractured site
d they help in maintaining the external rotation of the right leg

24.9 The countertraction provided in fixed traction is provided by:

a Jonathan's body weight
b suspending the splint from a balkan beam
c elevating the foot of Jonathan's bed
d tying the cords which extend from the skin extension to the end of the Thomas splint

24.10 Healing of bone in this type of fracture commences with:

a the deposition of calcium and phosphate in the fracture site
b callus formation
c haematoma formation
d osteoblast activity

25 Meniscectomy

PATIENT'S PROFILE

Arthur has always been a keen sportsman playing football, squash and cricket since his schooldays. Over the last two years he has been increasingly troubled by a knee which seems to 'swell' every now and then. It is not overtly painful but he canot bear his own weight and is forced to wear elasticated support around his right knee during any sport.

On the advice of the football club physiotherapist Arthur visits the orthopaedic surgeon who, after a detailed examination and a series of X-rays, advises Arthur he has a torn lateral meniscus of the right knee which will never repair and suggests that it should be removed if Arthur wants to continue being active in sports. Arthur is a professional cricketer, being regularly selected for the county team, and is keen to continue his cricketing career. He accepts the surgeon's advice and arrangements are made for Arthur to be admitted to hospital in six weeks time. In the waiting interval Arthur is advised to rest and continue to wear his elasticated knee support.

25.1 **A useful first aid measure during the 'swelling' of Arthur's knee would be to:**

a apply a hot compress
b apply a compression bandage
c massage the knee vigorously
d give an 'alcohol' rub

25.2 **Which of the following is the underlying cause of Arthur's torn meniscus:**

a twisting movement with the knee flexed and the foot on the ground
b rotation movement with the knee extended and the foot off the ground
c extending movement with the knee rotated and the foot on the ground
d flexion movement with the knee extended and the foot off the ground

25.3 The one procedure which should be greatly emphasized in Arthur's preoperative preparation is:

a giving prescribed prophylactic antibiotics
b grouping and crossmatching three units of blood
c toleration and endurance to physiotherapy
d arthroscopy and synovial fluid aspiration

25.4 Immediately following meniscectomy Arthur's affected limb should be positioned with the knee:

a flexed at 45°
b extended at 90°
c flexed at 90°
d extended at 0°

25.5 The surgeon instructs the nurse to apply a Robert Jones bandage to the affected knee. This type of bandage:

a supports an unstable joint
b gives the required joint immobility for 10 days
c prevents joint effusion
d maintains the circulation of a weakened joint

25.6 Following his meniscectomy Arthur should regularly exercise the group of muscles known as the:

a hamstrings
b gastrocnemius
c quadriceps
d gluteals

25.7 Arthur will be allowed to bear weight on the affected limb when:

a all joint stiffness has been overcome
b there is no risk of joint effusion
c the sutures have been removed
d the risk of infection no longer exists

25.8 Arthur is taught to raise the affected limb with a weight attached to the foot. This exercise increases the effort needed to:

a extend the muscles

b extend the knee

c contract the knee

d flex the muscles

25.9 Normally the knee joint gains its stability from the:

a junction of femur and tibia

b cruciate and lateral menisci

c articular surfaces

d limited range of movements

25.10 Prior to discharge Arthur is advised that:

a he will no longer be able to play active sports

b after a check in 4 weeks he should be able to take up sports again

c he should always wear a compression bandage when he is allowed to start playing sports again

d he can safely play squash and cricket but not football after he recovers

26 Laminectomy

PATIENT'S PROFILE

Joe Maddison had a 4-year history of back trouble. He could trace the origins of his problem to when he was thrown from a horse and had landed with considerable impact on his left side rolling over quickly to avoid the hooves of the horse. Ever since then he has had prolonged periods away from his office where he is an insurance broker.

The excruciating pain extends from the lower spine down the right leg and is severe enough to keep Joe immobilized for several days at a time. Over this 4-year period various treatments which have brought temporary relief include bedrest, traction, physiotherapy, heat therapy, analgesia and the wearing of a spinal corset. None of these treatments has resolved the basic problem of relieving the irritation of the spinal nerves as they enter and leave the spinal cord between the affected vertebra within which the nucleus pulposus has slipped.

When Joe was referred to the orthopaedic surgeon a series of X-rays were requested and these included a myelogram. After studying the X-ray results the surgeon advised Joe that the best treatment for his back trouble was a laminectomy which he proposed to perform in three weeks time if Joe was agreeable.

26.1 One form of treatment that Joe was given included traction for 1 month. The type of traction most likely to have been employed was:

a unilateral fixed skeletal traction
b unilateral Hamilton–Russell traction
c bilateral sliding skin traction
d bilateral fixed skin traction

26.2 The area of the spine in which intervertebral disc lesions are most commonly located is the:

a coccyx
b sacrum
c lumbar
d thorax

26.3 A myelogram would outline the:

a spinal theca
b meninges
c nerve tracts
d nerve roots

26.4 Pressure exerted on the right side of the spinal cord affecting the spinothalamic tract will affect any movement:

a on the right lower limb below the vertebral lesion
b on the left lower limb below the vertebral lesion
c bilaterally below the level of the vertebral lesion
d on the right limb above the level of the vertebral lesion

26.5 **Joe should be advised that the operation of laminectomy involves the removal of the:**

a body of the affected vertebra
b the nucleus pulposus
c posterior spinal processes
d lateral spinal processes

26.6 **Which one of the following terms implies the fusion of two joints:**

a arthroplasty
b arthrodesis
c arthrectomy
d arthrostomy

26.7 **Joe is nursed in the dorsal position for 24 hours postoperatively and after 18 hours he has not passed any urine. This is most probably due to:**

a spinal shock
b dehydration
c position
d spinal oedema

26.8 **Prior to being ambulant Joe should be encouraged to concentrate on:**

a leg-raising exercises
b quadricep exercises
c shoulder and arm exercises
d deep breathing exercises

26.9 **The joints of the vertebral column are mainly:**

a synarthrotic
b amphiarthrotic
c diarthrotic
d condyloid

26.10 **In advising a nursing colleague about the correct method of lifting a heavy object you would recommend that the body posture should be:**

a knees apart, elbows flexed, head upright, feet apart and spine straight

b elbows straight, spine flexed, head extended, feet apart and knees apart

c head flexed, feet apart, knees together, elbows straight and spine flexed

d feet together, knees together, elbows flexed, neck extended and spine straight

27 Congenital Dislocation of the Hip

PATIENT'S PROFILE

Mrs Purvis had an uneventful pregnancy giving birth to a baby daughter, Lucy, who weighed 4.5 kg. Having completed the initial screening tests the paediatrician referred Lucy to the orthopaedic surgeon who confirmed that she had a congenital dislocation of the right hip. The surgeon also noted that Mrs Purvis herself had suffered from the same problem when she was born.

Although anxious and disappointed Mr and Mrs Purvis accepted the situation and listened very carefully to the plan of care proposed by the surgeon. Lucy was to be cared for at home for the greater part of the period of treatment. Mrs Purvis would have to be shown how to put on double nappies and be counselled on the particular dangers associated with nursing Lucy in the prone position. The surgeon advised Mrs Purvis to breastfeed.

A health visitor would visit and check on how both Mrs Purvis and Lucy were coping, and would be available at any time if Mr and Mrs Purvis had any anxieties or problems. Arrangements would be made to see Lucy in the outpatients department at monthly intervals when the surgeon would check on Lucy's growth and development and decide if further treatments or investigations were needed.

Before Lucy reached the crawling stage it was proposed that she would be admitted to hospital for vertical Gallows traction, this to be immediately followed by a period of abduction traction. This treatment should reduce the femoral head into the acetabular socket. If successful it would then be followed by applying a Lorenz (frog) plaster for a prolonged period to maintain the reduction until Lucy achieved further growth and development.

27.1 The cause of congenital dislocation of the hip is:
- a due to a recessive trait carried by the mother
- b due to the child being born in the breech position
- c the subject of continuing research
- d due to a viral infection in the first trimester

27.2 The most comon finding related to congenital hip dislocation is that it is:
- a bilateral with a high incidence in girls
- b unilateral and more common in girls
- c bilateral with a high incidence in boys
- d unilateral and more common in boys

27.3 Diagnosis of congenital hip dislocation is confirmed by testing for:
- a Ortolani's sign before 7 days old
- b Trendelenburg's sign before 5 months old
- c Ortolani's sign before 7 months old
- d Trendelenburg's sign before 6 days old

27.4 In showing Mrs Purvis how to apply double nappies the nurse should explain to her that the extra thickness will:
- a limit the movement of the lower limbs
- b immobilize and support the pelvic girdle
- c provide greater abduction of both hip joints
- d increase the abduction of the left hip

27.5 **Lucy's weight at 3 weeks old increased to 5 kg and she was taking 5 feeds in each 24 hour period. Her daily fluid requirement per kg of bodyweight would be approximately:**

a 75 ml
b 100 ml
c 125 ml
d 150 ml

27.6 **Since Lucy was to be nursed in the prone position while at home Mrs Purvis would be strongly advised to:**

a ensure that Lucy's cot covers never go above her shoulder level
b start Lucy on bottle feeds as soon as possible
c avoid using any type of soft support for Lucy's head
d ensure that Lucy always 'burps' after each feed

27.7 **Mrs Purvis, on asking for advice on the prognosis of Lucy's future, is most likely to be told that:**

a Lucy would have to wait until her growth and development were complete until she achieved full mobility
b corrective surgery may have to be considered if Gallows traction and the Lorenz plaster therapy did not successfully correct the dislocation
c the outlook is promising since the diagnosis was made early
d Lucy would always have limited mobility since the hip socket was very shallow

27.8 **At 10 months old Lucy was admitted for Gallows traction for 15 days and abduction traction for 15 days. Two important features to check during vertical Gallows traction are that:**

a the buttocks rest carefully on the mattress and the foot of the cot is elevated
b traction cords are always taut and the weights free from any obstruction
c the buttocks are raised off the mattress and the head of the cot is elevated
d the buttocks are exposed and the limb bandaging reaches midthigh level

27.9 **At the completion of 15 days' abduction traction to reduce the hip dislocation the degree of abduction should be:**

a 90°
b 120°
c 140°
d 180°

27.10 **After the Lorenz plaster cast was applied and completely dried Lucy was discharged home. The nurse would advise Mrs Purvis that Lucy:**

a would require passive physiotherapy to all her limbs three times a day
b should be allowed to play freely and be as active as possible
c would need strict toileting to avoid soiling the plaster
d should be confined to her cot or play-pen for her own safety

28 Spinal Cord Injury

PATIENT'S PROFILE

Reginald, an 18-year-old trainee electrician, was given the task of securing electrical cable to an outer brick wall on the second level of a three storey building. When turning around on the scaffolding platform his foot missed the firm base and he toppled over the platform railing.

He fell six metres and in falling sustained a forceful impact to his back on a low level brick wall. His foreman and colleagues rushed to his assistance but were horrified when Reginald said he could not move or feel his legs. While they waited for the ambulance they kept Reginald warm but did not move him in case they made matters worse.

28.1 **When a spinal cord injury is suspected the first aid which the ambulance crew gives must include:**

a checking the lower limbs for their range of movement
b avoiding flexion and extension of the vertebral column
c turning the patient onto his right or left side
d giving analgesic anaesthetic, e.g., Entonox, to relieve pain

28.2 The initial local response to the injurious impact is:

a paralysis
b haematoma
c muscular spasm
d spinal shock

28.3 On admission to the ward Reginald was diagnosed as suffering from 'transection of the lumbar spinal cord'. This implies that:

a mixed neurones and autonomic pathways are possibly damaged below the site of injury
b motor and sensory neurones supplying the lower limbs are irreversibly damaged
c motor and sensory pathways are inhibited from reaching the cerebral cortex
d mixed neurones can no longer innervate the pelvic organs and lower limbs

28.4 The diagnosis was said to be provisional since Reginald was suffering from 'spinal shock' which masked the true neurological signs and symptoms. Spinal shock would be expected to last for:

a 12–24 hours
b 24–72 hours
c 4–7 days
d 2–8 days

28.5 Reginald complained of severe muscular spasm which did not abate with either analgesics or correct positioning. One procedure which would relieve the intolerable pain is a:

a lumbar vertebral manipulation
b laminectomy
c rhizotomy
d radiant heat therapy

28.6 To reduce the hazards of urinary incontinence Reginald was catheterized. His oral fluid intake was set at a target volume of 2.5 litres per 24 hours. This volume would prevent renal:

a calculi
b ischaemia
c necrosis
d thrombosis

28.7 After 2 weeks of being nursed in a Stryker frame, Reginald complained of profuse perspiration of the upper limbs and thorax. This diaphoresis is most probably due to:

a delayed emotional reaction to the injury
b damage to the heat-regulating mechanism in the hypothalamus
c increased bloodflow from the pelvis and lower limbs
d increased autonomic sympathetic activity

28.8 Reginald had no control over his bowel functions. To minimize faecal incontinence and establish a regular pattern of bowel evacuation it is recommended that Reginald:

a is given an evacuant enema every 3 days
b is given a bulking aperient each day
c has increased dietary fibre and extra fluids
d has a manual evacuation of the lower colon every 3 days

28.9 When Reginald is first introduced to a programme of wheelchair dependence the greatest danger to him is:

a injury to his lower limbs
b hypotension and fainting
c uncoordination of the upper limbs
d the hurting of injured vertebrae

28.10 In the long term, to give Reginald a positive social outlook it is useful to introduce him to:

a the disablement resettlement officer
b competitive sports
c the occupational therapist
d archery and javelin throwing

29 Fracture of the Ankle

PATIENT'S PROFILE

Sally, aged $15\frac{1}{2}$ years, thoroughly enjoyed sports and was school captain of the first hockey team. During practice, while making a running pass, she swerved to avoid impact with an opponent. In twisting her body, her foot stayed fast as she fell over. She suffered a sharp pain on the inner aspect of the left ankle and in falling over inverted the left foot. When helped to stand she could not bear any weight on her injured foot without suffering excruciating pain.

In hospital 30 minutes later her ankle had evidently become swollen and was hot and tender to touch. The X-ray showed a fracture which the surgeon decided required open manipulation under general anaesthesia followed by immobilization with a below knee plaster of Paris. Sally's parents could not be contacted as they were abroad visiting a sick relative. However, her elder brother accompanied Sally on her admission to the ward.

29.1 The first aid which could be recommended for Sally is:

a a cold compress to the injured ankle
b to remove the footwear and apply a compression bandage
c for her to lie still and to reassure her
d to secure the injured ankle to the opposite sound limb

29.2 The consent for general anaesthesia could be signed by:

a Sally
b Sally's brother
c the surgeon
d the anaesthetist

29.3 The doctor's notes indicate that Sally has suffered a Pott's fracture. This would imply that the bones most likely to be affected are the:

a talus and lower third of the tibia
b calcaneus and lower third of the fibula
c internal malleoli and lower third of the tibia
d external malleoli and the lower third of the fibula

29.4 The affected foot was extremely swollen, this being due to:

- a haematoma, ligament injury, oedema, and bruising
- b soft tissue injury, muscle spasm, and ligament injury
- c oedema, muscle spasm, haematoma, and tendon rupture
- d muscle spasm, haematoma, bruising and ligament tear

29.5 The foot has:

- a 8 tarsal bones forming the ankle
- b 7 carpal bones forming the ankle
- c 3 arches from talus to phalanges
- d 8 metatarsals forming the phalanges

29.6 The most common injury to the foot and ankle affecting teenagers in sport is a:

- a fracture
- b sprain
- c strain
- d dislocation

29.7 After manipulation Sally's casted limb is positioned on a firm pillow and elevated to a 45° angle which allows for:

- a good air circulation to dry the cast
- b venous bloodflow
- c correct alignment of the reduced fracture
- d observation of the extremities

29.8 The postoperative X-ray shows good bone alignment but Sally was advised she could not weightbear for 6–8 weeks. In this case Sally should:

- a become wheelchair dependent
- b learn to use crutches
- c have the heel of the plaster cast reinforced
- d attend physiotherapy 3 times a week for 6 weeks

29.9 Prior to her discharge from hospital Sally's cast should be checked for:

- a sensory response and movement of the toes
- b peripheral temperature and painful stimuli
- c cast shaping and contour
- d colour and temperature of the toes

29.10 Which statement correctly identifies the characteristics of the ankle. The lower end of the tibia and fibula articulates with the:

a talus, has hinge movement with dorsal and plantar flexion

b calcaneus, has gliding movement with flexion and extension

c talus, with cartilagenous movement and can abduct and adduct

d calcaneus, has synarthrotic movement providing dorsal and plantar flexion

30 Fracture of the Patella

PATIENT'S PROFILE

Agatha, aged 30, had a previous history of ulcerative colitis which made an excellent response to steroid and dietary therapy. She was receiving the final stages of her drug regimen when she was involved in a car crash. The collision caused her to hit the left patella on the car dashboard causing a linear fracture.

On admission to accident and emergency during the evening she produced her 'steroid card' and was able to give an accurate account of her drug dose for the colitis. This was:

prednisolone 20 mg twice daily for 7 days
15 mg twice daily for 7 days
10 mg twice daily for 7 days
10 mg twice daily for 5 days

She was now on the 23rd day of her steroid therapy.

After a physical examination and skeletal scan the surgeon confirmed the presence of a fracture and a profuse joint effusion. The treatment plan was as follows:

A full length plaster cast over a double padded left leg, which was to be bivalved after the cast had dried. The cast was then to be secured by firm crepe bandaging while Agatha remained on bedrest for 10 days.

A second full length cast was to be applied with the limb protected by a single layer of stockinette. This second cast would remain on for 6 weeks during which time Agatha could go home, having learned the correct use of crutches.

From her social assessment it was noted that Agatha lived alone in a second floor flat, but her sister would come and live with Agatha until she made a full recovery.

30.1 The amount of prednisolone Agatha had taken up to the point of admission was:

a 0.680 mg
b 6.50 mg
c 650 mg
d 680 mg

30.2 One of the long-term effects of prednisolone is to inhibit bone healing. This occurs because prednisolone causes:

a oedema
b osteomalacia
c hypokalaemia
d osteoporosis

30.3 Prednisolone is one of a group of substances referred to as steroids. More accurately prednisolone is a:

a synthetic glucocorticoid
b mineral corticoid
c adrenal medulla hormone
d natural glucocorticoid

30.4 Prednisolone hinders bone healing by:

a delaying haematoma formation
b disorganizing osteocyte activity
c interfering with calcium metabolism
d inhibiting callus formation

30.5 The first plaster cast was bivalved to allow for:

a correct alignment of the patella
b absorption of tissue fluid
c a defined period of bedrest
d promotion of bone healing

30.6 After admission to the ward Agatha insisted on a vegetarian diet. Which group of the following foods would ensure an adequate dietary intake of calcium:

a cabbage, rice, watercress and white flour
b fresh citrus fruits, pulses and potatoes
c bananas, carrots, rice and strawberries
d brown bread, lettuce, potatoes and tomatoes

30.7 While learning to use crutches Agatha tended to take her bodyweight on the axillae. This is a dangerous practice because it can cause long-term:

a hunching and stiffness of the shoulder girdle
b damage to the radial nerve and wrist drop
c cervical spinal stress leading to backache
d upward tilting of the pelvic girdle and coccyx

30.8 Agatha's sister should be advised that until the plaster cast is removed her most valued contribution would be:

a aiding Agatha with sitting into and rising from a chair
b helping Agatha in climbing up and down the stairs
c removing non-slip rugs from the flat
d assisting Agatha in her personal toilet and dressing

30.9 The single layer of stockinette applied to the limb would help to:

a counteract itching below the cast
b make the removal of the cast easier
c shape the contours of the cast edges
d minimize the pressure on the casted limb

30.10 The best action to promote comfort after the removal of the cast is to:

a apply a soothing oil to the skin
b dust the skin with a fine talcum powder
c wash the limb with hot soapy water
d assess the loss of muscle tone

Geriatric Case Histories

31 Pneumonia and Head Injury

PATIENT'S PROFILE

While cooking the evening meal Mrs Carter tripped over a loose kitchen tile and in falling severely gashed the skin over the temporal bone and lost consciousness for several minutes.

On arriving home her bachelor son found his mother in a conscious but shocked state, her face and clothing covered in blood. He immediately telephoned for an ambulance and then cleaned Mrs Carter's face and head as best he could.

In the accident and emergency department the wound was toileted and sutured under local anaesthetic. A skull X-ray showed no obvious bone injury and the initial neurological observations were all within normal limits. On taking Mrs Carter's previous medical history the physician noted that she had psychiatric treatment for periods of endogenous depression, and had been taking nitrazepam (Mogadon) for the last 6 years to overcome insomnia. He admitted Mrs Carter to the acute geriatric ward requesting 1-hourly neurological observations for the next 12 hours.

31.1 Which one of the following observations should be reported immediately if it occurs:

- a rising pulse rate and falling blood pressure
- b rising pulse rate and rising blood pressure
- c falling pulse rate and rising blood pressure
- d falling pulse rate and falling blood pressure

31.2 Although Mrs Carter's neurological observations remained within the normal limits she remained agitated and restless requiring a nurse to remain with her continuously. Her restlessness is most probably due to:

- a increased intracranial pressure
- b endogenous depression
- c Mogadon being omitted that evening
- d reactionary shock

When reviewed the following day Mrs Carter's axillary temperature was 39.6°C and her respirations were laboured and painful. The physician diagnosed bilateral lobar pneumonia and prescribed:

normal saline 0.9% 500 ml intravenously every 12 hours
ampicillin 500 mg intravenously every 6 hours
flucloxacillin 500 mg intravenously every 6 hours
chest physiotherapy
culture and sensitivity of a specimen of sputum
venous blood specimen to be taken for haemoglobin level

31.3 The causative organism of the pneumonia was identified as being *Staphylococcus pyogenes*. This organism is a:

a bacillus
b diplococcus
c pneumococcus
d bacterium

31.4 During the next 24 hours the physiotherapist treated Mrs Carter twice, the therapy of choice being:

a chest percussion and vibration
b postural drainage taping with fingers or light ham
c deep inhalation/exhalation exercises
d oropharnygeal suction

31.5 Forty-eight hours after the antibiotic therapy commenced, the X-ray showed no resolution of the pneumonia. The physician then prescribed probenecid (Benemid) 500 mg 3 times daily. This drug would:

a reinforce the affect of the ampicillin
b act as a bronchial dilator
c improve the blood levels of the antibiotics
d act as an anti-inflammatory agent in the lungs

31.6 Forty-eight hours after admission Mrs Carter's nursing care was gauged on the Norton Scale at 10, this implies that she was being nursed:

a at absolute bedrest
b for partial mobility
c as capable of self care
d at full mobility

31.7 The main characteristics of Mrs Carter's sputum are most likely to be:

a tenacious and rust-coloured
b viscous and purulent
c mucoid and watery
d frothy and white

31.8 Although recovering both from her head injury and the pneumonia it was noted that Mrs Carter's haemoglobin level was low enough to warrant 2 units of blood. In iron deficiency anaemia blood is, as a general rule, transfused when the haemoglobin level is from:

a 4–7 g/100 cm^3
b 8–10 g/100 cm^3
c 11–13 g/100 cm^3
d 13–18 g/100 cm^3

31.9 To overcome Mr Carter's anxieties about his mother coping on her own at home, the ward sister requested a home assessment. Those in the caring team who are best placed to perform this task are the:

a occupational therapist, health visitor, social worker, physiotherapist
b ward sister, district nurse, general practitioner, physiotherapist
c occupational therapist, ward sister, social worker, district nurse
d ward sister, general practitioner, medical aids department, social services

31.10 In her long-term interests Mrs Carter should be advised to:

a continue for several more weeks with physiotherapy in the outpatients department
b visit her general practitioner for an alternative hypnotic
c have a further opinion from a psychiatrist regarding her depression
d take the advice of the district nurse regarding safety in the home

32 Hypothermia

PATIENT'S PROFILE

Mr A Crawford, aged 76 and a widower living alone has been found by his neighbour 'in a collapsed and neglected state'. On examination the general practitioner advises that Mr Crawford should be admitted to the geriatric unit for assessment and treatment for hypothermia and malnutrition. Very little is known about Mr Crawford except that he has a married daughter living some distance away in a remote farming area.

32.1 **On his admission to the ward the most appropriate nursing position for Mr Crawford would be:**
a dorsal position
b prone position
c lateral position
d semirecumbent position

32.2 **Mr Crawford has no relatives living in the immediate locality. Which authority should take responsibility for his home while he is in hospital:**
a police
b local housing department
c social services
d hospital

32.3 **When undressing Mr Crawford the nurse finds his pension book in his trouser pocket. Who would normally accept responsibility for the safe custody of this personal property:**
a unit administrator
b unit nursing officer
c ward sister or charge nurse
d medical social worker

32.4 **In the initial phase of Mr Crawford's hypothermia his blood pressure is likely to be:**
a hypertensive
b hypotensive
c normotensive
d labile

32.5 **The most sensible nursing therapy to counteract Mr Crawford's hypothermia after undressing him would be to:**
- a give him a hot drink
- b cover him with a lightweight blanket
- c give him a warm bath
- d dress him in warm clothing

(reduce)

32.6 **Those nursing measures expected to be carried out upon Mr Crawford include:**
- a pulse, temperature, blood pressure, respiration and urinalysis
- b blood pressure, respiration, pulse, temperature and skin colour
- c respiration, pulse, temperature, blood pressure and chest X-ray
- d temperature, blood pressure, blood count, pulse and respiration

32.7 **After studying Mr Crawford's history which would be the nursing priority:**
- a to give a medicated bedbath because the skin is neglected and dirty
- b absolute bedrest for at least 24 hours
- c to consult the dietician regarding the correction of malnutrition
- d to contact Mr Crawford's daughter

32.8 **Mr Crawford will have recovered from his hypothermia when his rectal temperature reaches:**
- a 34–35°C
- b 36–37°C
- c 37–38°C
- d 38–39°C

32.9 **During the first 24 hours following recovery from his hypothermia, the most suitable dietary measure would be to give Mr Crawford:**
- a cool fluids only
- b an easily digested, light protein diet
- c measured amounts of liquefied food by nasogastric tube
- d a normal diet

32.10 Which of the following nutritional elements would promote a healthy skin:

a iron, protein, carbohydrates and vitamin D
b protein, roughage, water, vitamins A and C
c fats, minerals, proteins, vitamins A and B complex
d water, proteins, minerals, vitamins A and C

33 Cerebrovascular Accident

PATIENT'S PROFILE

Mr Halliday is a prosperous elderly shopkeeper who could also be regarded as a workaholic. Over the last few months he and his wife have been busy planning conversions to their shop with the idea of extending their range of goods.

During this time Mr Halliday tended to ignore recurring headaches. Eventually, however, when the headaches became severe he had to stop work and take rest periods. It was while resting that he lapsed into a coma from which his wife could not arouse him. The emergency doctor on call admitted Mr Halliday to hospital with a provisional diagnosis of cerebrovascular accident.

Several hours after his admission Mr Halliday has recovered from his coma but has a flaccid paralysis of both the right arm and leg. He is agitated because of an indwelling urinary catheter and does not appear to be able to focus properly.

33.1 Following his recovery from coma the most important nursing action would be to encourage Mr Halliday to:

a sit out of bed, comfortably positioned in an armchair
b move all limbs at prescribed intervals
c maintain the position of his limbs in the optimal anatomical position
d change his position every 4 hours to avoid the risk of pressure sores

33·2 The nurse observes that when approached from the right Mr Halliday is rather indifferent but when approached from the left is obviously aware of her presence. It may be correct to deduce that Mr Halliday's right eye is affected by:

a diplopia
b ptosis
c hemianopia
d photophobia

33·3 Apart from the nursing care given to Mr Halliday, which member of the caring team should be giving intensive therapy. The:

a occupational therapist assessing the aids required for daily living
b speech therapist in promoting better verbal communication
c ophthalmologist to correct the visual defect
d physiotherapist to improve locomotor coordination

33·4 Mr Halliday's urinary catheter is to be removed. To minimize the risk of postcatheterization incontinence the nurse should, prior to the catheter's removal:

a encourage Mr Halliday to do sphincter control exercises
b clamp off the urinary drainage tube for 2–4 hourly intervals
c give a bladder washout with an antibiotic solution to control infection risk
d ensure that the bowel is completely empty before removing the catheter

33·5 Mr Halliday's bedside locker should be positioned to his:

a left side parallel with his hand
b right side parallel with his elbow
c left side parallel with his shoulder
d right side parallel with his hand

33·6 The hemiplegia suggests that the blood vessel in the circle of Willis most likely to be affected is a branch of the:

a anterior cerebral artery
b middle cerebral artery
c posterior cerebral artery
d basilar artery

33·7 The senior of two nurses caring for Mr Halliday could set a professional caring standard to her junior colleague by:

a insisting on silence while giving physical care to Mr Halliday
b helping the junior nurse to feed Mr Halliday correctly
c teaching the junior nurse about cerebrovascular accidents
d ensuring that Mr Halliday's position is altered frequently

33·8 Mrs Halliday expresses concern that she will not be able to care for her husband and maintain their business concern. She could be advised that:

a she should consider selling the business since Mr Halliday will need 24-hour care.
b when finally assessed the health visitor will advise her of help available
c the general practitioner will visit very regularly, assess progress and prescribe care
d with daily visits to the outpatients department Mr Halliday will make good progress

33·9 Mrs Halliday asks the nurse what the future prospects are for her husband's full recovery. The best response to this enquiry would be:

a she should take advantage of all the help available for her husband's future
b if Mr Halliday persists with the physiotherapy he will make excellent progress
c once Mr Halliday is discharged from hospital his general practitioner will explain everything
d it is necessary for her to have an interview with the physician

33·10 The area of the brain most likely to be affected by the cerebrovascular accident is the:

a right hemisphere
b occipital lobe
c frontal lobe
d left hemisphere

34 Cataract

PATIENT'S PROFILE

Mrs Dawson, aged 68 and a widow, has of recent months found increasing difficulty with her vision, being unable to focus on peripheral objects. The general practitioner diagnosed a left cataract and also organized an outpatient appointment for Mrs Dawson to be seen by an ophthalmic surgeon. Agreeing with the diagnosis the surgeon suggested that the cataract should be removed by a lens extraction under local anaesthetic. He would admit Mrs Dawson as a day patient since there were no other physical considerations.

34.1 **Which one group of clinical features is Mrs Dawson most likely to complain of prior to her admission:**
- a excess tearflow, scleral redness, gritty feeling within the eye
- b severe localized pain and photophobia
- c iritis and irregular shape of the pupil
- d reduced visual field especially in daylight

34.2 **The most likely cause of Mrs Dawson's cataract is:**
- a irradiation of the cornea
- b degeneration of the lens
- c the use of contact lens
- d obstruction of the lacrimal apparatus

34.3 **A cataract interferes with vision because it:**
- a increases pressure within the vitreous humour
- b reduces drainage from the posterior chamber
- c alters the power of accommodation
- d prevents light reaching the retina

34.4 **Which procedure is essential before surgery takes place:**
- a temperature, pulse, respiration and blood pressure
- b urinalysis to exclude diabetes
- c height and weight to exclude obesity
- d conjunctival swabs to exclude infection

34·5 Prior to her operation Mrs Dawson should be told that after surgery she should:

a expect to have both eyes covered
b keep her head upright after the operation
c not open her bowels for 48 hours
d remain on bedrest for 24 hours

34·6 The surgeon prescribed syringing of the lacrimal duct before surgery. This procedure should:

a render the left eye surgically clean
b reduce the pressure within the anterior chamber
c promote natural tearflow across the sclera
d prevent the risk of conjunctivitis

34·7 Postoperatively the intraocular pressure can be markedly increased by:

a sudden head movement, speech and swallowing
b mastication, coughing and defaecation
c the dorsal position, speech and defaecation
d swallowing, sneezing and defaecation

34·8 On inspection of the affected eye after the operation, the nurse checks the:

a scleral incision
b iridectomy
c conjunctival incision
d lacrimal incision

34·9 Prior to her discharge Mrs Dawson would be advised to:

a keep the right eye covered for 6 weeks
b return to the outpatients department for removal of sutures
c return to the hospital in 6 weeks for a lens prescription
d continue her eye drops twice daily for 6 weeks

34·10 The normal shape of the eyeball is maintained by the:

a contents of the anterior chamber
b posterior chambers
c vitreous humour
d coats of the eye

35 Total Hip Replacement

PATIENT'S PROFILE

Mrs Gordon, a widow with a depressive personality, had been confined for the last 4 years to her ground floor council flat due to severe osteoarthritis of her right hip. Everyday activities such as dressing, cooking or shopping were impossible because of the very limited movement and painful stiffness locally and the wasting of the muscles of the right leg. Her two daughters visited regularly to care for her and also obtained the services of a home help twice a week and meals-on-wheels 3 times a week.

Mrs Gordon had over this 4-year period been taking analgesics (aspirin) and anti-inflammatory drugs with little effect. She had been on the waiting list for a total hip replacement for 2 years and was admitted for surgery 2 days before the scheduled operation. This was Mrs Gordon's first time in hospital and her daughter expressed some anxiety that her mother, although keen to have the operation, was extremely depressed.

35·1 **Total hip replacement surgery is a therapy which is a:**
- a prosthetic replacement of the head of femur
- b cup arthroplasty following acetabular reaming
- c arthrodesis of the acetabular and femoral head
- d acetabular arthroplasty and femoral head prosthesis

35·2 **Mrs Gordon, having a depressive personality, could be mentally stimulated in the preoperative phase by:**
- a permitting her daughters to visit at any time
- b encouraging her to join in ward activities
- c introducing her to a patient with a similar background
- d introducing her to a patient with a similar disease

35·3 **The underlying pathology of Mrs Gordon's illness can be described as being:**
- a infective
- b inflammatory
- c degenerative
- d autoimmune

35·4 Preceding the normal preoperative physiotherapy Mrs Gordon would receive instructions:

a in deep breathing exercises
b to strengthen the affected limb
c to strengthen the upper limbs and shoulders
d to achieve maximal movement of the pelvic girdle

35·5 Immediately following surgery the nurse would concentrate on preventing:

a pressure ulcers
b urinary retention
c hip dislocation
d chest infection

35·6 Mrs Gordon's wound is drained by a vacuum bottle. While this is in position it is most important to:

a ensure a small volume of antiseptic solution in the bottle
b support the bottle so that it is always below the wound level
c clamp off the drainage tubing before moving Mrs Gordon
d maintain Mrs Gordon in the semiprone position to ensure wound drainage

35·7 On checking the vacuum drainage the nurse notes there is no change in volume over a period of 3 hours. The nurse should then check the:

a drainage tubing is patent
b wound for any exudate
c antenna on vacuum bottle
d securing clip on the bottle neck

35·8 While she is confined to bed the position of the affected limb is maintained in:

a neutrality
b abduction
c adduction
d external rotation

35.9 **To maintain the desired position on the affected limb the nurse should:**

- a use a bedcradle to relieve the limb from weight of bedclothing
- b apply gentle skin traction for 48 hours
- c secure the limb position using sandbags
- d place a covered pillow between the patient's knees

35.10 **The most likely appliance to be issued to Mrs Gordon so that she would continue her physiotherapy at home is a:**

- a glide chair
- b wheelchair
- c walking frame
- d walking stick

36 Parkinson's Disease

parkinson drugs
BNF 181

PATIENT'S PROFILE

Alice, a widow aged 72, has now been resident in the geriatric unit for 23 weeks. The Parkinsonism from which she was suffering is now under reasonable control. Her past medical history revealed that she had suffered from a cerebrovascular accident 2 years ago and this left her with a residual minor contracture of the left elbow. Persistent sinusitis has caused partial deafness of the left ear for which she requires a hearing aid.

For over a year before admission Alice slowly developed the classical signs and symptoms of Parkinson's disease (paralysis agitans). She recalled how tired she always felt, and the more tired she was the more difficulty she had in controlling the tremors of her hands and legs, especially the tremor of her thumb and forefingers. Her back muscles were persistently stiff and combined with the cramp-like pain in her feet and calf muscles made her feel 'rigid' and incapable of movement. Immediately before her admission she became unsafe on her feet and could only achieve walking by shuffling slowly and using very short steps. Her two sons were more alarmed when they could not understand their mother's slow monotonous speech, noticed a constant dribbling of saliva and her stoop which became pronounced. On being told the diagnosis the elder son thought it best to sell off Alice's flat and use the money to pay for the residential care she would need for the rest of her life. This, as it turned out, was the main cause of Alice's depression.

The immediate investigations of chest X-ray, ECG and blood glucose levels all proved negative, and the physician prescribed:

diazepam (Valium) 2 mg three times daily for anxiety
temazepam (Normison) 10 mg at night for insomnia
carbidopa and levodopa (Sinemet) 274 mg twice daily

This drug regimen resolved many of the problems created by the disease with the minimum of side effects, eventually the sedative drugs were withdrawn. The nursing team from the outset aimed at relieving the problems created by Alice's depression, anxiety, lack of confidence, incorrect posture, loss of balance, incontinence, weight loss and overperspiration. Their success was measured by comparing the Norton Scale scored over the 23 weeks, this rose from 9 to 17. Alice is now physically and psychologically ready for Part III Accommodation.

36.1 In Parkinson's disease the chemical neurotransmitter which is deficient is dopamine and is secreted by the:

a corpus striatum and reacts with acetylcholine
b basal ganglia and reacts with noradrenaline
c substantia nigra and reacts with acetylcholine
d corpus callosum and reacts with noradrenaline

36.2 The classical symptoms of Parkinson's disease from which Alice suffered were:

a insomnia, weight loss, poor posture, and muscle rigidity
b bradykinesia, monotonous speech, fatigue and incontinence
c shuffling gait, stooping, incontinence and insomnia
d pin rolling tremor, muscle rigidity, bradykinesia, and poor speech

36.3 Sinemet helped to relieve Alice's rigidity, tremor and postural instability because the drug includes:

a a naturally occurring amino acid
b a precursor to dopamine
c the motor end plate neurotransmitter
d achieving a high serum level within 6 hours

36.4 With a Norton Scale of 9 the first measure which will encourage Alice to become mobile is for the nurse to:

a teach Alice in the use of a Zimmer walking frame
b increase Alice's periods of armchair rest each day
c encourage activities involving all muscle groups for 5 minutes every hour
d give passive massage of the limbs 3 times daily

36.5 In the early stages of treatment Alice had no confidence in herself or in the physiotherapy aids which would encourage her to be mobile. To introduce mobility it would be better to:

a teach Alice in the use of a wheelchair
b provide a 2 nurse escort each time Alice has a walk
c provide a nurse escort who will support Alice on her affected side
d introduce Alice to remedial hydrotherapy

36.6 The most valuable method of helping Alice regain her balance would be for the nurse to:

a ensure that all articles Alice is likely to require are within easy reach
b ensure that Alice sits squarely and upright when in bed or in a chair
c encourage high stepping exercises for five minutes 3 times a day
d make Alice aware of her body posture by the use of a full length body mirror

36.7 Alice was incontinent of urine at the time of her admission. In the absence of any functional disorder this problem could initially be overcome by:

a taking Alice to the toilet every 2 hours
b ensuring that a commode is positioned by the bedside at all times
c offering a bedpan every two hours
d passing a catheter until she becomes mobile

36.8 In the early stage of drug therapy Alice perspired very profusely at the slightest exertion. To make Alice more comfortable the nurse could:

a give Alice a bedbath twice daily
b ensure that Alice wears loose fitting cotton clothes
c provide a multidirectional fan at the bedside
d encourage Alice to use a body deodorant

36.9 The greatest hazard to Alice throughout her chronic illness will be:

a joint contractures
b bone injuries
c infection risks
d pressure ulcers

36.10 Part III Accommodation implies that Alice will be offered:

a a single person's ground floor flat from the local housing authority
b a warden controlled ground floor flat located in the hospital grounds
c a single person room in a health authority nursing home
d shared accommodation in a warden controlled nursing home

37 Residential Care

PATIENT'S PROFILE

Mrs Edna Ferguson, 78, a widow for the last 10 years, was admitted to the geriatric unit for residential care while her spinster daughter had a 4 week holiday. Miss Ferguson, before going on holiday, gave the nursing staff a detailed profile of her mother's needs. From this information the staff gathered that Mrs Ferguson:

was independently self caring and a cheerful personality
had partial deafness of the right ear for which she wore a hearing aid
wore spectacles, one pair for reading, a second pair for distance vision

tended to constipation
suffered from insomnia with a tendency to get out of bed in the middle of the night.

Miss Ferguson left three telephone numbers where she could be contacted in case of emergency and said she would telephone her mother each morning at 11.00 hours. Within a few days of her admission the nursing staff discovered that Mrs Ferguson had faecal impaction and noted that she was becoming increasingly withdrawn.

37.1 **Which one of the following is the most effective method of dealing with Mrs Ferguson's sensory deprivation:**
a assess the effectiveness of the hearing aid and spectacles
b familiarize Mrs Ferguson with the unit and members of staff
c reassure Mrs Ferguson that she will be well looked after
d position her bed near to the nursing observation station

37.2 **Mrs Ferguson's periods of confusion at night are most probably due to:**
a arteriosclerosis
b faecal impaction
c environmental disorientation
d dreaming and retrospective memory

37.3 **The nursing diagnosis of faecal impaction is based upon:**
a abdominal distension and borborygmi
b fetid breath odour and constipation
c spurious diarrhoea and constipation
d disinterest in diet and withdrawn behaviour

37.4 **To resolve faecal impaction the first nursing measure would be to:**
a administer evacuant enemata every day for 3 days
b administer an olive oil retention enema
c increase the dietary fibre and daily fluid intake
d manually evacuate the lower bowel contents

37·5 Mrs Ferguson would wake up about 02.00 hours and, in some confusion, try to get out of bed, talking in a confusing and rambling fashion. The first nursing action should be to:

- a check that the upright security bed rails are correctly secured
- b offer to take Mrs Ferguson to the toilet
- c address Mrs Ferguson by name
- d switch on the bedside light

37·6 In settling Mrs Ferguson for the remainder of the night the nurse should pursue the following sequence of events:

- a adjust both the bedclothing and Mrs Ferguson's position, offer toilet facilities
- b reassure Mrs Ferguson, give a warm drink with a prescribed sedative
- c offer toilet facilities then give sedation with a warm drink
- d offer toilet facilities, adjust bedclothing, reassure and offer a warm drink

37·7 Toilet facilities should always be offered to Mrs Ferguson before she is settled for sleep because of her:

- a faecal impaction
- b environmental confusion
- c sensory deprivation
- d cerebral changes

37·8 Mrs Ferguson's withdrawn behaviour could be countered by mentally stimulating her by:

- a assisting her to pursue personal hobbies
- b introducing her to occupational therapy
- c encouraging her to participate in small group activities
- d telephoning her daughter every day at 11.00 hours

37·9 Which quality of sound is improved by a hearing aid:

- a clarity
- b frequency
- c pitch
- d volume

37.10 To ensure that Mrs Ferguson gains the most benefit from her hearing aid the nurse would check that the:

a right auditory canal is free of cerumen
b microphone is worn over the top clothing
c amplifier sits comfortably above the pinna
d right tympanic membrane is free of cerumen

38 Rehabilitation Programme

PATIENT'S PROFILE

Mrs Young, aged 72, although twice widowed was a cheerful personality and for the last 2 years had been a resident of an old people's home. The nursing officer in charge of the home thought that Mrs Young was an excellent candidate for rehabilitation at the local geriatric hospital and asked for the geriatrician's opinion.

For over 10 years Mrs Young had suffered from the complications of arteriosclerotic disease. A mild cerebrovascular accident had left her with a minor residual right hemiplegia for which she wore a brace on the right lower limb. In addition she had what was thought to be aphasia but on further investigations turned out to a dual receptive and expressive dysphasia made worse by a slight facial paralysis. There was a history of hypertension and heart failure, both under reasonable control with the following therapy:

methyldopa (Aldomet) 5 mg 3 times daily
digoxin (Lanoxin) 0.0625 mg once daily
frusemide (Lasix) 40 mg once daily
bumetanide (Burinex) 2 tablets daily

Since her stroke Mrs Young had been catheterized with a self-retaining Foley catheter which was used to overcome problems of incontinence and potential risk of pressure ulcers. There was a partial deafness of the left ear due to Ménière's disease which Mrs Young had suffered some 20 years previously.

After a case conference the caring team agreed to accept Mrs Young into the rehabilitation programme and set their objectives as being:

restore urinary continence within 7 days of removing the urinary catheter

restore maximal mobility within 2 weeks of commencing special physiotherapy exercises
commence a course of speech therapy which would be ongoing for 12 months
return Mrs Young to her residential home within 6 weeks.

38.1 **A rehabilitation programme should take into account the patient's 'self image'. Which of the following would positively encourage Mrs Young to take some pride in her personal appearance:**

a ensure that she has a hair shampoo at least once weekly
b her wearing a suitable dress to disguise her leg brace
c give constant reminders of how smart she appears
d remove the self-retaining Foley catheter

38.2 **To help Mrs Young reconstruct her body image to one of normality the most helpful nursing action would be to:**

a reinforce and praise existing abilities
b encourage activities with others in her peer group
c introduce her to a self-help therapy clinic
d evaluate the nursing objectives each week

38.3 **Mrs Young had some perceptual loss and a short span of concentration so the nurse should aim at preventing self injury by:**

a encouraging Mrs Young to ask for help as and when needed
b promoting self awareness of residual disability
c teaching the patient to walk correctly
d encouraging manipulation and movement of the right arm

38.4 **When Mrs Young is trying to express herself verbally, the nurse could usefully help her by:**

a encouraging socialization with other patients
b evaluate verbal skills for any improvement
c listen carefully to anticipate any special needs or wants
d encourage the use of common core language expression

38.5 **Expressive dysphasia refers to:**

- a responding correctly to verbal stimuli received by the temporal lobe
- b the correct use of facial muscles to pronounce words
- c non-response to verbal stimuli due to partial deafness
- d responding incorrectly to verbal stimuli collated by the frontal lobe

38.6 **Receptive dysphasia refers to:**

- a responding incorrectly to verbal stimuli received by the temporal lobe
- b inarticulate responses due to facial muscle paralysis
- c non-response to verbal stimuli due to partial deafness
- d responding incorrectly to verbal stimuli collated by the frontal lobe

38.7 **After removing the urinary catheter and, bearing in mind the objective stated by the caring team, the nurse should:**

- a despatch a specimen of urine for culture and sensitivity
- b check the undergarments for urinary soiling every 2 hours
- c irrigate the bladder with a mild antiseptic solution
- d establish the pattern of expected incontinence

38.8 **Damage to the 7th cranial nerve will usually result in:**

- a partial deafness
- b aphasia
- c facial paralysis
- d visual deterioration

38.9 **The pathology of Ménière's disease progresses to:**

- a degeneration of the acoustic nerve
- b sclerosis of the ossicles of the middle ear
- c trauma to the cochlea and labyrinth
- d vertigo and perceptive deafness

38.10 Mrs Young's right ankle and foot tended to avert and this would normally be corrected by:

a ensuring that the correct size and width of shoe is worn
b placing the affected foot into the inverted position at frequent intervals
c assessing the suitability of the leg appliance
d ensuring that Mrs Young attends arranged remedial physiotherapy classes

39 Acute Monocytic Leukaemia

PATIENT'S PROFILE

Mrs Bates, aged 73, a widow for the last 8 years lived with her bachelor son in a ground floor council flat. She had suffered from a stroke over 2 years ago but had made an excellent recovery from this and now coped reasonably well with the triple handicap of cataract, partial deafness and incontinence of urine. Her son was very supportive and dealt with the housekeeping and shopping although he also worked full-time.

Her sudden admission to the general hospital was due to a dramatic episode of epistaxis which lasted for 48 hours and required a transfusion of 20 units of blood. When this crisis was contained a more detailed examination revealed haematuria and extensive purpura. A bone marrow puncture confirmed a suspected diagnosis of acute monocytic leukaemia.

Mrs Bates was transferred to the acute ward of the geriatric unit to deal with her established handicaps and was prescribed the following antileukaemic regimen:

prednisolone (Predsol) 20 mg 3 times daily
cytosine arabinoside, or cytarabine (Cytosar) 60 mg daily for 5 days by subcutaneous injection
thioguanine (Lanvis) 60 mg twice daily for 5 days
daunorubicin (Cerubidin) 40 mg daily by intravenous injection until further instruction

The nursing plan included care for the following problems which were ascertained after taking a careful nursing history:

haemorrhagic episodes
ankle oedema
urinary incontinence
immobility
iron deficiency anaemia
dehydration
poor nutritional state
prone to infection

39.1 **The antileukaemic drug regimen induced a remission of the symptoms. This would imply that:**
a a permanent cure has been achieved
b routine blood tests would now show normal values
c the acute features of the disease have been arrested
d Mrs Bates can now have radiotherapy to the granulocytic tissues

39.2 **An acute monocytic leukaemia implies that the blood investigations would reveal:**
a a neoplastic proliferation of immature granulocytes
b an excessive neoplastic proliferation of lymphocytes
c increased cellularity of the bone marrow
d the loss of normal immune responses

39.3 **The haemorrhagic episodes of haematuria, purpura and epistaxis, which are symptomatic of leukaemia, are due to:**
a decreased production in the erythropoietic tissues
b decreased production of the coagulation factors
c increased permeability of the capillaries
d inadequate reserves of and inadequate dietary iron

39.4 **Which of the following drugs is a pyrimidine antagonist to the mutated DNA/RNA in the cancer cell:**
a daunorubicin
b thioguanine
c cytarabine
d prednisolone

39.5 **In addition to being reverse barrier nursed to protect Mrs Bates against cross-infection hazards, she was also given a powerful antibiotic called:**

a daunorubicin
b thioguanine
c cystosine arabinoside
d prednisolone

39.6 **The tendency to haemorrhagic episodes was partially controlled by the drug:**

a daunorubicin
b thioguanine
c cytarabine
d prednisolone

39.7 **Mrs Bates had a cystometric examination which revealed a residual volume of 210 ml of urine. This result would infer that she:**

a should persist with continence therapy which has a good prognosis
b should be temporarily catheterized until she regains mobility
c requires to be permanently catheterized to avoid pressure ulcers
d has urinary retention with overflow due to bladder neck obstruction

39.8 **The ankle oedema should clinically resolve when:**

a the legs are elevated to assist venous return
b the iron deficiency anaemia is treated with iron compounds
c oral fluids are restricted
d the antileukaemic therapy is concluded

39.9 **Which one of the following would be of the greatest psychological benefit after the drug regimen is completed:**

a measures to control altered bowel habits
b provision of a wig because of alopecia
c provision of a Zimmer frame to promote mobility
d referral to the occupational therapy department for assessment

39.10 Mrs Bates' son is most likely to be advised by the physician that his mother's expected prognosis is:

a an expected lifespan of no longer than 12 months
b an expected lifespan between 3 and 5 years
c a normal lifespan unless there is a relapse
d frequent relapses which will respond to treatment

40 Terminal Illness

PATIENT'S PROFILE

Mr John Dobson, a widower, at the rather young age of 64 was terminally ill. He was suffering from an inoperable cancer of the left lung and metastases of the lumbar spine. Three weeks ago he was admitted to the ward for the chronically sick in the geriatric unit because neither of his 3 married daughters could give the intense nursing care he now required.

His medical regimen was palliative, aimed at relieving his symptoms of chest pain, immobility, nausea, dysphagia and insomnia. For these he was prescribed:

Brompton Hospital Cocktail 15 ml as required with a daily review of the dose
chlorpromazine (Largactil) 50 mg three times daily
temazepam (Normison) 10 mg at 22.00 hours each evening

The medical notes indicated 'all nursing care' and excluded resuscitation as a possible nursing measure. The nursing team aims were set to meet Mr Dobson's physical, psychological, spiritual and social needs. A major problem for Mr Dobson was the emotional turmoil he experienced just before and for 1 week after his admission. The symptoms of his cancer were under good control and in the last 2 weeks of his life the aims of nursing care were achieved, his death was quiet and dignified with his 3 daughters at the bedside.

40.1 **Which of the following groups shows the most likely sequence of emotional reactions which Mr Dobson suffered once he realized he could be dying:**

a rejection, denial, anger, acceptance
b denial, rejection, anger, acceptance
c anger, denial, rejection, acceptance
d acceptance, anger, rejection, denial

40.2 **Mr Dobson reacted with great hostility to medical and nursing staff during the first 2 days in hospital. Nurses should understand that anger in the terminally ill patient is:**

a triggered off by abrupt and over officious staff
b an expression of anxiety to altered body image
c one means of obtaining sympathy to his distress
d a self recognition that no cure is possible

40.3 **For several days Mr Dobson refused his medication and his carefully planned diet. Such a refusal indicates that the mental defence mechanism being used to cope is:**

a projection
b rejection
c denial
d anger

40.4 **Mr Dobson tires very easily spending a great deal of time resting. In his best interest his daughters should be advised to:**

a visit at any time but for short periods only
b visit at set periods each day for no more than 30 minutes
c liaise with the nurse regarding the best visiting times
d discuss with Mr Dobson the best time to visit

40.5 **Brompton Hospital Cocktail contains:**

a morphine, whisky, procaine, sucrose, chloroform
b cocaine, brandy, honey, morphine, sucrose
c rum, ethyl alcohol, morphine, honey, choloroform
d gin, chloroform, cocaine, morphine, honey

40.6 Who of the following is best placed to advise Mr Dobson to put his legal affairs in order:

a eldest daughter
b lawyer
c physician
d ward sister or charge nurse

40.7 Mr Dobson's employer arrives unexpectedly and asks to see him, but Mr Dobson refuses to see this visitor. The nurse should:

a refer the employer to the physician
b advise the employer that Mr Dobson is asleep and cannot be disturbed
c asks the employer to visit later when Mr Dobson is more amenable
d refer the employer to Mr Dobson's eldest daughter

40.8 In the medical notes Mr Dobson is referred to as being 'cachexic'. This term implies that he has:

a gross spinal deformity
b extreme muscular wasting
c severe chest symptoms
d inoperable cancer

40.9 Twenty-four hours before dying Mr Dobson exhibited Cheyne–Stokes respiration. This means that there was a period of:

a prolonged apnoea followed by rapid respirations
b sighing respirations followed by cardiac dyspnoea
c paroxysmal respirations followed by apnoea
d cardiac dyspnoea followed by sighing respirations

40.10 A junior nurse on duty at the time of Mr Dobson's death was emotionally upset. Her senior colleague should:

a send her off duty until the following day
b give the junior nurse 5 minutes privacy to collect herself
c make her a cup of tea and offer some sympathy
d ask her to help in preparing for last offices

Answers

Medical Case Histories

1 Pernicious Anaemia

ANSWER SHEET

1.1 c Although tired, Mrs Drobney would not be physically exhausted (**a**) after a period of bedrest. Peripheral anoxia (**b**) would show as a cyanosis and is not reflected in the case history. Transfusion of packed cells (**d**) would raise the blood pressure since it adds to the circulatory volume and increases blood viscosity.

1.2 c The extrinsic factor (**a**), i.e., Vitamin B_{12}, is available in the average diet. In the absence of the intrinsic factor, however, it cannot be absorbed in the ileum and thereafter utilized for the production of erythrocytes, hence the anaemia. Gastrin (**b**) and hydrochloric acid (**d**), if absent, are not replaced by intramuscular injection.

1.3 b All intramuscular injections can be painful (**a**) and carry a risk of sciatic nerve injury (**d**). If the skin is stained (**c**) the injection has been given too superficially.

1.4 a The metric symbol for microgram is μg. Its prefix is 10^{-6}, and its multiplication factor is 0.000 001.
milligram = mg = 10^{-3} = 0.001
nanogram = ng = 10^{-9} = 0.000 000 001
picogram = pg = 10^{-12} = 0.000 000 000 001

1.5 d Vitamin B_1 is aneurine; vitamin B_2 is riboflavine; vitamin B_6 is pyridoxine and is closely related to vitamin B_{12}.

1.6 b Erythroblasts are immature red blood cells or erythrocytes; leucocytes are white blood cells and thrombocytes, also known as platelets, are involved with natural coagulation.

1.7 b Schilling test is a radioactive test using cobalt to measure the uptake of vitamin B_{12}. Snellen's test is used to discriminate visual acuity; Schiller's test detects the presence of cancer of the cervix and Schlesinger's test is to indicate the presence of urobilinogen.

1.8 a Since the absence of the intrinsic factor is lifelong, replacement therapy by one injection every 4–6 weeks is absolutely essential to prevent the recurrence of the symptoms of pernicious anaemia.

1.9 c This is a rare complication nowadays, but if it does occur the mixed nerves entering and leaving the spinal cord become partially demyelinated. This leads to a wide variety of both sensory and motor neurone damage ultimately leading to lower limb paralysis.

1.10 c The bone marrow (**a**), especially of long and some flat bones are the site of production, but not the site of storage of mature erythrocytes. The pancreas (**b**) is irrelevant to the question. The spleen (**d**) often acts as a 'reservoir' organ storing blood for short periods of time.

2 Chronic Bronchitis

ANSWER SHEET

2.1 b This is the only reason for 'requesting' a specimen of sputum. Options **a**, **c** and **d** are visual observations which are valuable when assessing Mr James' progress on a day to day basis.

2.2 a Oxygen is a dry gas and if it is prescribed for prolonged use it will readily dry the bronchial mucosa and prevent the other options from occurring effectively. Therefore humidification is essential.

2.3 c The term *broad spectrum* means wide-ranging. Antibiotics are not directly effective against viruses precluding options **a** and **d** from being correct.

2.4 **b** Frusemide (Lasix) does not act within the glomerular apparatus, being most efficacious on the ascending loop of Henle.

2.5 **c** Once absorbed through the rectal mucosa into the bloodstream, aminophylline is taken to and acts directly on the bronchial muscle. The muscle is relaxed allowing the diameter of bronchial lumen to dilate; once this occurs **a** and **b** will occur. Option **d** is irrelevant.

2.6 **b** Intravenous therapy (**a**) given to an oedematous patient would add to the problem. Oral toilet (**c**) must be offered at regular intervals because of the oxygen therapy and the tendency to rely on oral breathing. Two litres of fluid per day would not compensate for the massive diuresis which is to be expected from frusemide, and could lead to **b** occurring.

2.7 **b** During a dyspnoeic attack the heart fails to pump an adequate volume of blood to the periphery. The peripheral temperature falls and the blood vessels constrict. This leads to poor gaseous exchange, hence cyanosis. While options **a**, **c** and **d** may exist, of themselves they are not the cause of cyanosis.

2.8 **b** The combination of oral breathing and oxygen therapy tend to dry the mucosa of the oral cavity (buccal cavity) making the tissues prone to infection. See also answer 2.6.

2.9 **a** In measuring vital capacity of the lungs the patient is asked to take a deep breath and then exhale forcefully into a flowmeter, e.g., Wright's Peak Flowmeter. The average normal range is between 400 and 600 litres of air per minute. Option **c** describes tidal volume, **a** is supplemental volume and **d** is irrelevant.

2.10 **c** Patients such as Mr James have an irreversible loss of alveoli, not only as a consequence of chronic bronchitis but with each acute respiratory tract infection. They are extremely prone to such attacks especially in the late autumn and winter months. The increasing loss of alveoli is partially overcome by the greater respiratory effort which leads to dyspnoea.

3 Myocardial Infarction

ANSWER SHEET

3.1 c The blood pressure and pulse (**a**) are guidelines only to the actual state of the heart at any given time; they would not determine if there was any risk when first mobilizing Mr O'Brien. The prothrombin time (**b**) is used to determine the dose of anticoagulants and raised cardiac enzymes (**d**) such as SGOT and SGPT take 7–10 days to return to normal levels. Whether the cardiac rhythm is determined by continuous monitoring or by daily electrocardiogram an abnormal trace indicates a further period of 24 hours bedrest.

3.2 d Either the apex beat or the radial pulse are counted, and if below 60 beats per minute the digoxin is withheld until a senior colleague has been consulted. As the digoxin improves the ventricular contraction and thus the cardiac output the blood pressure (**a**), pulse volume (**b**) and fluid balance (**c**) should improve as a consequence of the effect of the drug.

3.3 c Prochlorperazine (Stemetil) is an antiemetic (**d**), diamorphine (Heroin) is primarily used as an analgesic (**b**), and digoxin (**a**) is a cardiac glycoside. Regardless of which anticoagulant has been prescribed the patient's urine should be routinely ward tested daily for the presence of blood.

3.4 b Any circumstance which prolongs the prothrombin time increases the tendency to haemorrhage, e.g., anticoagulants or biliary obstruction and vitamin K should be readily available in the ward stock-cupboard. Protamine sulphate (**a**) is the specific antidote to heparin. Adrenaline and vitamin B_{12} are irrelevant.

3.5 c Options **a**, **b** and **d** are all predisposing factors to an actual necrosis of part of the heart muscle. A major difference is that while necrosis is irreversible, the other options can be reversed with suitable treatment.

3.6 c Option **a** is an assumption; **b** shows a lack of professionalism being a negative attitude to offer a patient's relative who may be distressed; **d** while optimistic is also an assumption. It should be appreciated by nurses that telling someone not to worry carries with it the implication that there is something to worry about and by so doing they increase anxiety levels.

3.7 b Regardless of the stage of training it is the duty of all learners to keep senior staff informed of changes in any patient's condition. If option **c** is selected it would indicate that the nurse has little or no appreciation of the severe unremitting nature of cardiac pain. Options **a** and **c** follow upon option **b**.

3.8 c In the long-term interest of the patient his closest relative would be the individual best placed to influence the patient's habits. This teaching and advisory role, however, begins in the hospital and medical and nursing staff should never underestimate the regard with which their advice is esteemed.

3.9 b The best way to control cholesterol (**a**) carbohydrate (**c**) and fats (**d**) all of which contribute to heart disease is to start by reducing the calorie intake. Many obese patients are started on a 1000 calorie diet while in hospital, and later this can be adapted to the individual's lifestyle when he or she is discharged from hospital.

3.10 b Minor haemorrhages (**a**) are the consequence of over dosage of anticoagulants. The clotting time of blood (**d**) involves assessing coagulation factors other than prothrombin. Option **c** is irrelevant.

4 Congestive Cardiac Failure

ANSWER SHEET

4.1 a The congestion refers to an impeded bloodflow through the cardiopulmonary circulation due to failure of both right and left ventricles. Pulmonary emphysema (**b**) would be a contributory factor if it were referred to in the case history. Blood pressure (**c**) at the periphery is usually low, and an incompetent aortic valve (**d**) would give rise to left ventricular failure.

4.2 **b** Fluid loss or gain is most accurately determined by body weight. A rapid gain or loss of 1 kilogram equals 1 litre of fluid. The remaining options are guidelines to the patient's progress.

4.3 **b** While the main effect of a diuresis is to rid the body of excess fluids a possible side effect is a reduction in the blood levels of potassium. Should these levels fall below normal values hypokalaemia may result, the danger then being a risk of cardiac arrest. To avoid this potassium chloride is given as a replacement therapy to maintain the potassium values between 3.5 and 5.3 mmol (3.5 and 5.3 mEq) per litre.

4.4 **c** Digoxin should be withheld if the pulse rate falls below 60 beats per minute because of the danger of heartblock, and then only given on the advice of the physician. Options **b** and **d** would follow in order of priority.

4.5 **c** A urinary diuresis should always be timed to occur during the day when nursing staff are best able to cope with the patient's needs for frequent toiletting. Equally the patient should be allowed the chance of natural sleep without the distress of toiletting. Options **a**, **b** and **d** are incorrect statements.

4.6 **b** Sodium chloride (table salt) has a natural affinity for water and therefore would worsen the tendency to oedema. While it is unpalatable to offer food in which salt has not been added in the cooking, commercial sodium-free salt is available for adding to prepared dishes. Glucose (**c**) being a sugar is a mild diuretic, animal fats and cholesterol (**d**) while limited would not directly influence the oedema. Potassium (**a**) is found in many fruit juices and would not influence the oedema.

4.7 **b** The primary cause of nausea in congestive cardiac failure is the congestion which also occurs in the gastrointestinal system.

Once treatment has commenced it may well be that the drugs could create a feeling of nausea (**c**).

4.8 a Normally the osmotic pressure of proteins exceeds that of the venules, which contributes to osmosis. When the pressures are reversed there is a pooling of tissue fluids at the capillaries. Option **c** is partially correct but it should be noted that arteries and veins are not exchange vessels therefore oedema does not actually occur around these vessels but at their tributaries, i.e., venules, arterioles, and capillaries.

4.9 a Mrs Morgan is to be nursed in a cardiac bed. Such a bed allows for the head of the bed to be elevated and the lower end to be tilted downwards creating an armchair effect.

4.10 a The failing muscle of a congested heart is very liable to an infarction, which follows upon a coronary thrombosis. Pulmonary embolism (**b**) can occur within the cardiopulmonary circuit but is more rare. Peripheral blood pressure (**c**) is usually low while option **d** is a partial repetition of the patient's diagnosis.

5 Asthma

ANSWER SHEET

5.1 c The upright position is absolutely essential to enable as much air as possible to enter and escape from the lungs in the extreme respiratory effort required during an asthmatic attack.

5.2 d The more severe asthmatic attack can give rise to cerebral anoxia. As the alveolar gaseous exchange is reduced the oxygen reaching the brain is also reduced, hence anoxia, followed by drowsiness. Options **b** and **c** can occur from the outset. Darren's pulse rate (**a**) was 140 beats per minute on admission therefore there has been an improvement.

5.3 **b** The histamines released from the irritated bronchiole cells have a constricting effect on the muscles of the bronchial lumen. Options **a** and **c** follow after the initial attack. Option **d** arises from the impulses sent from the respiratory centre located in the medulla oblongata.

5.4 **c** The extrinsic factor responsible is the protein found in the animal fur which initiates an intrinsic response. Emotional response (**b**) is not a proven initiating factor since an emotional response could well be the consequence of a natural predisposition to asthma. Genetic predisposition is not proven except to say that allergies such as asthma tend to be familial.

5.5 **c** Peak flow readings can only assess the volume of expired air and oxygen is only one of the gases exhaled. In children of Darren's age the average peak flow reading is in the range between 200 and 400 litres of air per minute.

5.6 **c** Oropharyngeal suction (**a**) and chest physiotherapy (**d**) are mechanical methods, and antibiotics (**b**) do not necessarily make infected sputum less viscous.

5.7 **b** The Inspiron oxygen mask mentioned in the history is a 'sealed' mask, i.e., it has no perforations in its structure which permit pure oxygen to mix with atmospheric air. The initial aim of the therapy would be to give a high concentration of pure oxygen to restore normal blood oxygen levels as rapidly as possible, best achieved in the short term by the use of a sealed mask.

5.8 **d** Chlorpromazine (Largactil) is the only sedative drug mentioned. Aminophylline (**a**) and salbutamol (**c**) are bronchial dilators while adrenaline (**b**) is a cardioneurogenic stimulant.

5.9 **d** Options **a** and **c** are impractical suggestions. There is nothing in the history to suggest that Darren is allergic to house dust (**b**).

5.10 **c** The pharmacological effect of Intal is to prevent the further release of histamine from irritated and damaged cells. It cannot deal with existing circulating histamines (**a**) and (**b**). Desensitization (**d**) is a therapy of gradual exposure to increasing levels of a causative allergen or irritant until the individual is no longer sensitive.

6 Deep Vein Thrombosis and Pulmonary Embolus

ANSWER SHEET

6.1 **a** Ibuprofen (Brufen) is derived from propionic acid and is usually prescribed for painful conditions **not** accompanied by a severe inflammatory disorder.

6.2 **d** When compared to a standard conversion chart Michael is overweight by 22 kg (48 lb) for his height. This is in excess of 10% of his desirable weight of 73 kg (161 lb) and he is therefore obese.

6.3 **a** The circulating macrophages will eventually liquefy the thrombus but this mechanism is only successful if the heparin prevents the blood clot from enlarging. Therefore **b** is the result of option **a**. Administered heparin does not influence the liver's ability to boost naturally occurring heparin (**c**) which is a plasma protein. Prolonging the bleeding time (**d**) is an undesirable side effect which may lead to minor haemorrhages.

6.4 **b** Acetylsalicylate acid (Aspirin) is well known for causing gastric irritation and it also prolongs the effect of heparin thus increasing the risk of gastric haemorrhage.

6.5 **c** TED stockings or elasticated hosiery are most effective on the superficial veins of the leg. They do, however, have a beneficial effect on the deeper veins (**b**) which would help to resolve the oedema (**a**) and may contribute to resolving **d**.

6.6 **d** Popliteal veins are superficial to popliteal arteries (**a**). Impeded bloodflow (**c**) does not indicate if it refers to venous or to arterial vessels, and option **b** is a possibility but not a certainty.

6.7 **c** The inferior vena cava is a major vessel conveying venous blood from the lower limbs and abdomen to the right atrium. The 4 pulmonary veins (**a**) are in fact arteries conveying oxygenated blood from the lungs to the left atrium. The superior vena cava (**d**) conveys venous blood from the head, neck and upper limbs to the right atrium. The iliac and hepatic veins (**b**) do not travel together, the former is found in the pelvis while the latter supplies the liver.

6.8 **d** The alcohol intake is too low to be considered relevant (**b**) and although the blood pressure (**c**) is within normal limits the diastolic pressure is slightly elevated. An idiopathic cause (**a**) suggests a natural predisposition in the absence of any other contributing factors. See also answer 6.2.

6.9 **d** A venogram requires that Michael be suitably attired in an operating gown and he may require some sedation (**a**). Option **b** is an incorrect statement and general anaesthesia (**c**) would be most unusual.

6.10 **d** General practitioners do not usually have facilities in their health centres or practices to carry out prothrombin blood tests (**a**). Prolonged rest periods (**b**) are inadvisable if the venous bloodflow requires stimulation by moderate exercise. While on a stabilized dose of warfarin it is not advisable for Michael to work in case of inadvertent injury and serious risk of haemorrhage (**c**).

7 Hypertension

ANSWER SHEET

7.1 **b** The analgesics mentioned in the options **a**, **c** and **d** do not correlate with the case history.

7.2 **c** Alcohol is not mentioned in the case history excluding options **a**, **b** and **d** from being correct.

7.3 **b** The T segment of the cardiac complex reflects the electrical conductivity resulting from ventricular relaxation. It can, however, also be distorted in hypokalaemia, ischaemia, ventricular hypertrophy, bundle branch block, and when digoxin is being used as a drug therapy.

7.4 **b** The diastolic pressure, i.e., the lowest pressure that is recorded by a sphygmomanometer relates to the relaxation phase of the cardiac cycle. It is often more important than the systolic pressure since a high diastolic pressure may indicate hypertension and this in turn may seriously impair the effective function of organs such as the heart, brain, kidneys and arterioles.

7.5 **a** The first morning specimen is always discarded because it contains a considerable amount of cellular casts and debris which may give a false reading when the total 24 hour specimen is assayed. Vanillylmandelic acid is only one of several end-products of adrenaline metabolism.

7.6 **a** Methyldopa (Aldomet) will lower high blood pressure by decreasing the resistance of the arterioles when the sympathetic nervous activity is reduced. In its metabolism it is reduced to methyldopamine, then methylnoradrenaline which is more persistent than naturally occurring noradrenaline. Once the blood pressure is reduced there is a subsequent fall in cardiac output.

7.7 **b** In such a short period of 48 hours the weight loss can only be attributed to the effect of the diuretic frusemide hence the increased secretion and excretion of urine. A massive diuresis in itself does not necessarily mean that the hypertension (**d**) is responding to therapy.

7.8 **d** The nursing role in this situation is always to refer the patients to their physician. Once the physician is convinced that patients understand the implications of discharging themselves then the nurse can proceed to the other options.

7.9 **a** Blood viscosity, i.e., the stickiness of blood is determined by the plasma proteins, in particular, albumen. The arterioles, also known as the resistance vessels, maintain a higher pressure than the arteries. As the blood flows from a wide diameter artery into a smaller diameter arteriole there is a mechanical resistance to bloodflow.

7.10 **c** Cholesterol (**a**), carbohydrates (**b**) and fats (**d**) will all be reduced if the calorie intake is controlled. Equally important is the method of cooking, e.g., frying and roasting are contra-indicated if fats are to be reduced and this advice is also important to Mr Arnold's wife who probably does the cooking.

8 Mature Onset Diabetes

ANSWER SHEET

8.1 **b** Pruritus or itching of the skin is a common symptom of mature onset diabetes. Petechia (**a**) refers to discoloration created by the bruising of small superficial blood vessels often seen on the dorsal surface on the hands of the elderly. Psoriasis (**c**) is a skin disease while polydipsia (**d**) refers to an excessive thirst which can only be relieved by drinking very large volumes of fluid and is a symptom of diabetes.

8.2 c Insulin (**a**) would utilize any circulating glucose giving a false result. Options **b** and **d** are possible but not essential since they would not influence the test results.

8.3 a Option **b** is proven by liver function tests. The ability of the intestine (**c**) to absorb glucose is proven by the xylose test. The pancreas (**d**) secretes **not** excretes insulin.

8.4 c A normal individual's blood glucose tolerance level should not exceed 5 mmol per litre, but as Mrs Arundel is a diabetic this will be proven by an expected glucose curve peaking to 9 mmol per litre.

8.5 a Where 1 is followed by the symbol % it simply means 1 in 100.

8.6 b There is a difference between being overweight and obese. By contrasting the body weight with the height and comparing it to a standard chart, if the weight is 10% over the ideal then that person is obese.

8.7 d It is remarkable how high the systolic pressure can rise before there is evidence of heart failure (**c**) especially if the rise is of a transient nature. However, in diabetes the patients are more prone to arterial diseases such as arteriosclerosis of the peripheral and end arteries. Options **a** and **b** are irrelevant.

8.8 b Thirty per cent of patients taking chlorpropamide have an alcohol intolerance if alcohol is combined with the drug. Vertigo and headaches (**c**) can and do occur but much more rarely. Since chlorpropamide is effective for 20–40 hours, hypoglycaemia is a remote possibility. Option **a** is irrelevant.

8.9 d The major long-term complication of arteriosclerosis and changes in the bone structure of the feet cannot be overemphasized and this hazard is minimized from the earliest opportunity by correcting bad habits or teaching new attitudes regarding the care of the feet.

8.10 b As yet there is no research which positively gives a genetic link (**a**). Mature onset diabetes does not occur spontaneously (**c**) and the relationship between a viral infection and the onset of diabetes is often remarked upon but it is conjecture if it is coincidental or cause.

9 Juvenile Onset Diabetes

ANSWER SHEET

9.1 **b** A glycosuria of 2% will imply that there are 2 g of glucose in every 100 ml of urine. This deposit will raise the specific gravity of urine above its normal value of 1001–1030 even when the urine is typically excessive in volume and pale in colour.

9.2 **b** This first injection of insulin has caused a rapid utilization of glucose by the cells and reduced the blood glucose levels causing hypoglycaemia. Options **d**, **c** and **a** would occur in that order if the glucose drink was ineffective.

9.3 **c** At cellular level insulin enables glucose to cross the cell membrane and promotes the transit of amino acids and potassium. How insulin activates the receptors on the target cells is still uncertain. Option **a** is an incorrect statement. In juvenile diabetes there is an absolute lack of insulin in the pancreatic beta cells (**d**). The pancreatic alpha cells (**b**) secrete the hormone glucagon, which in normal healthy subjects regulates the effects of naturally occurring insulin and releases liver glycogen as glucose so limiting the unpleasant effects of a naturally occurring hypoglycaemia.

9.4 **c** Option **a** occurs in hypoglycaemia. A bounding pulse (**b**) occurs in hypoglycaemia and an irregular pulse is found in diabetic coma. Abdominal pain (**d**) is a remote possibility in hypoglycaemia but abdominal reflexes are absent in diabetic coma.

9.5 c Option **a** equals approximately 10 g, a dextrose tablet contains 10 g (**b**) giving a total of 20 g. To give 200 ml of diluted orange juice (**d**) is too vague to accurately calculate its gram content. 300 ml of milk equals 15 g and a level tablespoon of glucose weighs 15 g (**c**).

9.6 c As a guideline the average diabetic diet consists of:

Carbohydrate	40% =	180 g × 10 =	1800 calories
Protein	15% =	67 g × 4 =	268 calories
Fats	45% =	202 g × 10 =	2020 calories
	100%	449	4088

NB 1 g carbohydrate = approximately 4 kcal (17 kJ)
1 g protein = approximately 4 kcal (17 kJ)
1 g fat (unsaturated) = approximately 9 kcal (38 kJ)

9.7 a A temporary illness such as diarrhoea, vomiting or pyrexia places extra demands on carbohydrate metabolism and the glucose is utilized much more readily. The body fat and protein will then be used to produce a new energy source. To reduce this hazard the insulin is usually increased by 1 mark or 1% until the temporary illness is over. Under no circumstances should diabetic patients omit their insulin especially when suffering an intercurrent illness.

9.8 c From a medical point of view regular self-administration of the prescribed insulin is more important than the subtleties of the injection technique itself. Options **a**, **b** and **d** are more often than not accepted as the nursing role in the education of a diabetic patient.

9.9 c The oxidation of fat in the absence of glucose leads to the formation of toxic substances such as ketones.

9.10 d A constantly high blood sugar, e.g., 10 mmol per litre, is beyond the physiological renal threshold for glucose, and at such a high level the sugar acts as a diuretic hence the symptom of polyuria and subsequent loss of bodyweight.

10 Gastroenteritis

ANSWER SHEET

10.1 c Options **b** and **d** include some of the features of gastroenteritis, i.e., diarrhoea and vomiting but not weight loss which is a critical feature. Option **a** is most unusual, the fontanelles do not usually bulge in dehydration.

10.2 c If possible an infant's temperature should be recorded at the rectum (**b**); the exception to this being irritation, infection or inflammation of the rectal mucosa. Oral temperatures (**a**) are never taken in infants. It is possible to take the temperature at a skin crease (**d**) but the result is unreliable.

10.3 a *Escherichia coli* is a commensal organism to the host but if transmitted can become pathogenic to the infected person, hence the need for very strict hygiene in handling infant's feeds. *Proteus vulgaris* (**b**) is more likely to be the causative organism of skin infections. *Candida albicans* (**c**) is the causative organism of thrush while *Treponema pallidum* (**b**) causes syphilis.

10.4 c In all children's wards the policy should be that of free visiting and, if required, overnight accommodation for the parents. Therefore the parents should arrange their visiting times with the nurse in charge of the ward. This policy serves to maintain the child–parent bonding.

10.5 c Paediatric drugs are prescribed mainly by the child's weight although the other options, **a**, **b** and **d**, are considerations in the overall plan of therapy.

10.6 a The calculation is determined by knowing that there is 250 mg in 1 ml which is divided by the dose, i.e., 62.5 mg, the answer being 4 or $\frac{1}{4}$ of a millilitre which is 0.25 ml.

10.7 b By adjusting the feeding bottle at the correct tilt the teat can be kept full thus preventing the infant from swallowing air.

However, in most cases a little air is swallowed necessitating the infant to be burped halfway through and at the end of each feed.

10.8 d Sodium hypochlorite 1%, sodium chloride 16.50% (Milton 1 in 80) is the usual antiseptic lotion used in the majority of homes and is recommended for both washing-up nursery utensils and for soaking feeding utensils for a minimum of one hour.

10.9 b If the child is being correctly isolated and nursed in a cubicle then the disease will not be airborne (**a**) to the main ward. It is most unusual and undesirable for children to share food (**c**) and the preparation of milk feeds is normally carried out within the strictest standards of hygiene determined by the Control of Infection Officer (**d**). When a nurse is caring for an infant with gastroenteritis under no circumstances should that nurse be giving direct personal care to other children.

10.10 c Along with other vital centres located in the medulla oblongata is that for vomiting, and the emphasis should be given to the phrase *coordination*. At the same time the cerebrum (**b**) is aware of the sensation and feeling created by vomiting, and the cerebellum (**a**) will adjust the muscular posture to allow for vomiting. The pons varolii (**d**) is a bridge of nerve fibres connecting the right and left cerebellar hemispheres.

Surgical Case Histories

11 Pyloric Stenosis

ANSWER SHEET

11.1 **d** After a nurse has given the infant a portion of the test feed, the paediatrician would palpate the junction of the stomach and duodenum to detect if there is a bulging of the pylorus. Options **a**, **b** and **c** would not of themselves contribute to a diagnosis of pyloric stenosis.

11.2 **c** A Billroth operation (**a**) refers to gastric surgery, Heller's operation is surgery which corrects achalasia of the lower third of the oesophagus, while Whipple's operation is reconstructive surgery of the head of pancreas where it enters the duodenum.

11.3 **c** A vertical incision into but not through the muscle layers of the pylorus allows the narrowed lumen of the pylorus to bulge open. When sutured horizontally the wider diameter is maintained.

11.4 **b** Copious and projectile vomiting leads to a loss of hydrochloric acid and gastric-secreted minerals. Such a loss, if excessive, permits the alkalis to exceed their normal values with an increase in the pH of blood above 7.4.

11.5 **d** Stagnant food tends to remain in the stomach despite the vomiting, and this debris gives rise to a gastritis, which is a localized inflammation. Vomiting (**a**), dehydration (**b**) and toxaemia (**c**) are problems giving rise to a generalized deterioration throughout the body.

11.6 **a** This defect is present from birth, i.e., it is congenital, but may remain asymptomatic until adulthood when the muscular weakness is exacerbated by heavy lifting or persistent coughing as in chronic bronchitis.

11.7 a Gastritis (b) is an inflammation of the gastric mucosa not an infection. Pyrexia (c) is a symptom of an underlying disease and toxaemia (d) is a general term indicating a toxic state which may be caused by either inflammation infection, allergic reactions, drug reactions, poisoning, etc.

11.8 a Occasionally during surgery the gastric submucosa is accidentally nicked creating a small connection between the stomach and the peritoneal cavity. This perforation will usually heal rapidly and a non-irritant solution of glucose saline, especially if boiled before being given and in a very small quantity, will not be hazardous to the infant. Glucose (b) is absorbed via the gastric mucosa but not in significant amounts. The carbohydrate content (c) is also true but the calorific value is so small that it is not significant until after the first 3 hours. Aspiration (d) is usually performed after each hour for 4–6 hours regardless of the oral feed prescribed and this aspiration will help with the initial healing of the anastomosis.

11.9 d Preoperatively the infants will usually guzzle their food impatiently and hungrily. Postoperatively, if the surgery has been successful, normal feeding can be resumed fairly quickly and the infant becomes contented. A bowel motion (a) if passed in the first 36 hours is most likely to be abnormal. If the intravenous therapy (b) is discontinued it indicates that fluid balance and intestinal motility are normal, not that the surgery has necessarily been successful. A gain in body weight (c) is certainly a good sign but there would not be any significant gain within 36 hours.

11.10 c The paediatric liaison officer (d) would probably contact the health visitor who should then arrange a series of visits to see how Timothy is progressing over the following fortnight. The general practitioner (b) will be advised by letter of Timothy's operation and will be available for a consultation if this is required. Only occasionally will a district nurse become directly involved with advising and counselling the parents of an under 5 year old.

12 Partial Gastrectomy

ANSWER SHEET

12.1 **c** Ulceration of the gastric mucosa occurs invariably on the posterior wall of the stomach which is related to the lesser curvature. Option **d** is more likely to be affected by a hiatus hernia or oesophageal varices. The greater curvature (**a**) of the stomach benefits from mucus-secreting cells which buffers the mucosa against the effect of hydrochloric acid. Rarely ulcers affect the actual junction of the pylorus and duodenum; they are, however, more likely to be affected by scarring and stenosis.

12.2 **d** A warning, skilfully and sympathetically given, that there will be postoperative pain creates a positive approach enabling the patient's coping mechanisms to deal with pain and therefore reduces the need for prolonged use of potent analgesia. Options **a**, **b** and **c** are vital but these are observations still subject to research appraisal.

12.3 **c** The main effects of atropine are to diminish the secretions of all exocrine glands with the exception of breast milk and to dilate the pupil of the eye (**a**). To relax involuntary muscle, which may induce drowsiness (**d**), reduces vagal tone thereby increasing the heart rate (**b**).

12.4 **c** The upper nasal cavity (**a**) is not influenced by the act of swallowing, and, without an advance warning, to start swallowing the tip of the tube would be an irritation to the pharynx (**b**) causing a gagging reflex. Without swallowing the tip of the tube may come to rest in the mouth when it reaches the oropharynx (**d**).

12.5 **b** Heller's operation (**a**) is a surgical repair of the lower third of the oesophagus for achalasia. Gastrojejunostomy (**c**) is an anastomosis between the greater curvature of the stomach and the jejunum. A vagotomy and pyloroplasty (**d**) is a surgical division of the gastric branch of the vagus nerve to reduce the volume of hydrochloric acid, and a reconstruction of the pylorus to increase its diameter.

12.6 d For a few hours after surgery the line of anastomosis may bleed very slightly, such blood being altered by the gastric secretions before it is aspirated.

12.7 c Secretions adhering to the inner or outer surface of the nasogastric tube may inadvertently find their way into the trachea and bronchus if the tube is removed without due care. The removal is preferably performed slowly with the patient in the upright position.

12.8 d Diaphragmatic spasms (hiccoughs) are due to irritation of the phrenic nerve which may be due to either the surgical procedure or the anaesthetic method.

12.9 a Dumping syndrome can occur from three causes: gross distension of the duodenal loop as food passes into it instead of onwards into the intestine; bile which may accumulate in the proximal loop created by the anastomosis or an excessive intake of carbohydrate into the intestine without sufficient gastric breakdown. This last cause may give rise to hypoglycaemia. Patients recovering from partial gastrectomy **must** have smaller meals and preferably have a rest before eating their main midday and evening meals.

12.10 a Options **b**, **c** and **d** are contributing factors which exacerbate a pre-existing condition, i.e., prone to excess secretion of hydrochloric acid which is not adequately buffered by sufficient mucus.

13 Inguinal Hernia

ANSWER SHEET

13.1 **b** Herniotomy (**a**) is a surgical incision into the neck of hernial sac to relieve an irreducible hernia and is often mistakenly referred to as a herniorraphy. A hernioplasty (**c**) is a plastic reconstruction for a radical repair of a hernia, i.e., Gallie's operation. Their is no such word as herniocele (**d**).

13.2 **c** Options **a**, **b** and **d** are all contributory factors to a pre-existing congenital weakness.

13.3 **d** A femoral hernia (**a**) is more common in women. An umbilical hernia (**b**) is more commonly seen in infants, while a ventral hernia (**c**) is a protrusion through the linea alba which is the tendinous junction running down the midline of the body from the xiphisternum to the pubis and being the blending of the oblique and transverse abdominal muscles.

13.4 **b** Options **a**, **c** and **d** are consequent upon the incarceration, i.e., a trapping of the peritoneal contents in the neck of the hernial sac.

13.5 **d** A respiratory spasm is a brief constriction of the involuntary muscles of respiration which in the majority of cases responds to an adjustment of the patient's position, e.g., from dorsal to lateral or vice versa. Oxygen (**a**) should be on hand for use after the spasm is over; the pulses (**b**) will be checked but would not resolve the respiratory spasm, and upward pressure of the lower mandible (**c**) ensures the tongue is brought forward and this will be helpful on recovery from the spasm.

13.6 **d** Surgical repair of inguinal hernia often causes retention of urine and for a male patient the natural posture for micturition is the best method of relieving what can be a most distressing complication. Option **a** is only going halfway in resolving the problem and is often a cruel reminder of the patient's distress. Option **c** is a useful psychological trigger if combined with option **d**. Option **b** will depend on the surgeon's postoperative instructions.

13.7 c On coughing the thoracic muscles and diaphragm contract raising the pressure within the abdomen which in turn exerts pressure on the wound. It is useful if, during coughing or lifting, the patient can exert a downward palm pressure on the wound which often overcomes a natural anxiety that the wound will 'burst open'.

13.8 c Within the inguinal canal lies the spermatic cord which of necessity may have been handled during the course of surgery. There may therefore be a secondary effect on the scrotal sac which may not only be painful but also slightly swollen. Options **a** and **b** are most unlikely in herniorraphy. Postoperatively patients may be reluctant to evacuate their bowel (**d**) because of indirect pressure on the wound, but this problem should have been anticipated in the preoperative phase.

13.9 c At 17 kg overweight (37 lb) there will be a definite stress to the integrity of the wound after the sutures have been removed.

13.10 a An overweight patient plus lifting heavy objects might well give rise to either a recurrence of the inguinal hernia or the risk of an incisional hernia. This is also related to answer 13.9.

14 Intestinal Obstruction

ANSWER SHEET

14.1 d The majority of intravenous fluids are administered to match the normal biochemical composition of body fluids. Isotonic fluids therefore maintain cellular osmosis, hypertonic solutions (**a**) increase osmotic pressure, and hypotonic solutions (**c**) decrease osmotic pressure. Option **b** is irrelevant.

14.2 d The term *hypovolaemia* refers to a reduction in the circulatory volume, hence a low blood pressure and a further exacerbation of shock. Hypovolaemia also implies a reduced circulatory volume to the kidneys hence oliguria.

14.3 d Option **a** is the responsibility of the surgeon or a member of his team, it is the duty of the nurse to 'check' that consent has been obtained. Options **b** and **c** can be completed once the premedication has been given.

14.4 a The patency of the transfusion can be threatened if the connection between the tubing and the intravenous cannula becomes detached during the movement of the patient from stretcher to bed.

14.5 b Potassium chloride would, in the first instance, be given to maintain the normal level between 3.5 and 5.3 mmol per litre, otherwise there is a serious risk of cardiac arrhythmias which precede a cardiac arrest.

14.6 c The surgeon would, in fact, be the best person to answer this enquiry, but as often as not, the nurse is asked the question. A knowledge of the surgeon's techniques would be helpful in this situation. In general terms a 'temporary' colostomy implies that at a later date there will be a permanent closure of the stoma under elective conditions, i.e., planned surgery when options **b** and **d** have been resolved. Option **a** is irrelevant.

14.7 b A colostomy appliance is designed in two main parts, i.e., the stoma seal and a drainage bag. It is undesirable to remove the stoma seal too frequently during the first few postoperative days, whereas the bag should be changed as frequently as is required. In regaining intestinal motility a great deal of flatus is produced which will inflate the colostomy bag unless it is pinholed on its upper edge to release the flatus.

14.8 c The stoma membrane is, in fact, insensitive to the touch and to applied pressure, hence the need to be careful when fitting the stoma appliance since undue pressure will not be complained of. The integrity of the stoma lumen (**b**) is active otherwise there would be no need for the nurse to be cleaning the stoma. It is very likely that there will be wound drainage (**d**) but this is secondary to the greater threat to the skin from excoriation by digestive enzymes and the potential to allergic reaction from any adhesives used.

14.9 d Oedema of the stoma (**a**) should have resolved by the third postoperative day. The odour (**b**) will remain a constant problem until the stoma is acting regularly and the best possible appliance has been chosen. The site of the colostomy (**c**) is an advantage to the promotion of formed faeces once the stoma is acting regularly.

14.10 b The basic principle in crossmatching blood is the matching of the recipient's plasma antibodies (serum) with the antigens in the proposed donor's blood cells. This is most accurately done using the indirect Coombs' test.

15 Ileostomy

ANSWER SHEET

15.1 b Written consent implies the patient has been 'informed', preferably by the operating surgeon as opposed to the consultant (**d**), who may only be referring the patient. Option **a** would be done after the consent form has been signed. The anaesthetist (**c**) would normally confine his expertise to the problems and risks associated with anaesthesia.

15.2 d High residue foods, e.g., cellulose (**a**), being bulky, increase intestinal motility and aggravate both the diarrhoea and the inflammatory condition. A low protein diet (**b** and **c**) would be inappropriate since a sound nutritional state depends on a rich supply of amino acids derived from protein from which to rebuild and repair damaged tissues.

15·3 a The lower colon should be washed out with warm tap water twice a day until there is a clear return ensuring that faecal and mucoid debris are removed. An enema saponis (**b**) is irrelevant in someone prone to diarrhoea; prednisolone retention enemas (**c**) are used as a conservative measure to promote healing of the mucosa of the lower colon. Sulphamethizole (**d**) is mainly used for infections of the urinary tract and should not be confused with the sulphathiazole, sulphadiazine and sulphamerazine often used to sterilize the gut.

15·4 c Vitamins A, C and D are derived mainly from a dietary source. While they can be temporarily stored in the body they cannot be synthesized from other materials from within the bowel.

15·5 c Once intestinal motility returns in the postoperative stage the stoma will expel digestive enzymes excreted from the intestinal mucosa and pancreas. A colostomy tends to expel flatus in the early stages postoperatively (**b**). Digested food is not a feasible option (**a**) since the patient is most likely to still be on a fasting regimen. Once intestinal motility has returned the activity of an ileostomy is very erratic, emptying on reflex stimulus.

15·6 b Pancreozymin and cholecystokinin are hormones released by the gastric mucosa. Hydrochloric acid and protease, being gastric enzymes, are most likely to be utilized before reaching the duodenum. Cholesterol and mucin are not digestive enzymes.

15·7 c A state of protein balance exists when there is an equilibrium between anabolism (tissue growth and repair) and catabolism (destructive metabolism). This is another way of saying that the amount of nitrogen in the body derived from protein foods equates the amount of nitrogen excreted in catabolic waste, e.g., the urea found in urine and faeces. When protein catabolism exceeds anabolism the patient is losing an excessive amount of nitrogen and this is what will happen in excessive loss of ileal fluid. The protein is broken down but is lost from the body before it can be utilized for tissue repair and growth.

15.8 c An ileostomy is a mutilating operation parallel with mastectomy, amputations or colostomy. Often the implications arising out of the altered body image to the patients and their relatives are not fully appreciated until the reality dawns in the postoperative phase. As a consequence the emotional turmoil varying from depression, frustration, aggression and anger are only a few of the coping mechanisms available to the patients to help them through the new situation.

15.9 c Following a colectomy vitamins B and C are not synthesized, as they were formerly, by the bowel. A light diet will not provide an adequacy of these vitamins to promote healing, hence the need for supplements during the convalescent period.

15.10 c Option **a** is not true. Unlike a colostomy the ileostomy tends to be erratic in its activity. Options **b** and **d** are relevant but are secondary to the major consideration of keeping the skin surrounding the stoma free from excoriation.

16 Ventricular Septal Defect

ANSWER SHEET

16.1 c The diagnosis of ventricular septal defect refers to a 'hole' in the septum separating the right and left ventricles. This defect permits a mix of arterial and venous blood, hence the expression *blue baby* which describes the resulting peripheral cyanosis. The ventricles will not empty correctly because the 'hole' alters the pressure within the ventricles preventing the valves from closing completely.

16.2 c Option **a** would be a popular choice except that a dentist would not be able to eradicate the organism *Streptococcus viridans*. Only a course of antibiotics would effectively rid the body of this organism. Orthodontic development (**b**) is considered well before the 'teething' stage. Loose teeth (**d**), if present, would be a possible hazard during anaesthesia.

16.3 c Neuroleptoanalgesia is a state of cooperation, sedation and analgesia induced by droperidol, one of a group of drugs used in anaesthesia. Dissociative anaesthesia (**a**) is a profound state of analgesia accompanied by a light sleep. Anxiolytic sedation (**d**) is induced by minor tranquillizers, e.g., the benzodiazepines. A state of euphoria and sedation (**b**) is a contradiction of terms.

16.4 a No comment is required on what should be a simple interpretation of anatomical terminology.

16.5 a The carotid artery (**d**) would not be a popular choice, not only because of its inadequate diameter to deal with the volume of blood returned to the body, but also because of its site. The pulmonary artery (**c**) is in fact a vein, and option **b** mentions 2 arteries when only one is to be cannulated.

16.6 c The right and left coronary arteries (**a** and **d**) are the principal supplies of oxygenated blood to the myocardium and they branch directly from the aorta. The pulmonary veins (**b**), which are 4 in number, are in fact arteries returning oxygenated blood to the left atrium but which are bypassed with the cardiopulmonary machine.

16.7 b Ventricular tachycardia implies fibrillation in which the ventricles will be unable to empty properly during the contraction phase which is extremely erratic. Tachycardia and/or fibrillation of the ventricles predispose to cardiac arrest. The quickest methods of restoring normal cardiac rhythm is to defibrillate the ventricles by passing a small voltage current through the organ. Option **a** is a temporary measure until defibrillation can be attempted. Options **c** and **d** would perhaps accompany or follow the defibrillation procedure.

16.8 a On restoring the circulation through the heart, the greatest risk will be coagulation in the coronary arteries, i.e., a thrombosis may occur at the time. Option **b** will be a risk once the chest wall has been closed. Sinus arrhythmia is to be expected and will be monitored for in the postoperative 48 hours. Collapse of the lung (**d**) should not occur if an underwater seal chest drain is established and maintained for the 48 hours following surgery.

16.9 d The metabolic needs (**a**) will be met by the prescribed intravenous therapy. Paralytic ileus (**b**) is a minimal risk since there has been no surgery on the gut. There should be minimal aspirate (**c**) from the stomach but the aspiration will keep the stomach deflated of 'gas' and reduce any tendency of upward pressure against the diaphragm and the heart.

16.10 c One-quarter or 25% of 3000 millilitres is 750 ml.

17 Splenectomy

ANSWER SHEET

17.1 a The simplest definition of *shock* is a fall in the blood pressure, but this response arises from a multiple sequence of events occurring within the body involving neurogenic reflex and biofeedback mechanisms. There is no such classification as vasomotor or primary shock (**b**), at the time of admission there is no clear evidence of haemorrhage (**c**) and the patient's blood pressure is normal at the time of admission (**d**).

17.2 b This radiating pain is also known as *referred pain*. For some as yet unknown reason the *visceral pain* is referred to as a surface area remote from the origin of the injured site and now becomes a *somatic pain*.

17.3 a The haematocrit compares the volume percentage of all the erythrocytes within 100 ml of whole blood. The ratio should be 45% cells to 55% plasma. Any variation from these figures would suggest a possible haemorrhage. It is a useful investigation in conditions such as burns, anaemia, haemorrhage from any cause, and the ratio of cells to plasma is usually raised in those living at high altitudes.

17.4 **b** This is an extension of the problem of shock, hence the need to keep very accurate records of pulse and blood pressure. Intraperitoneal bleeding (**a**) cannot be seen as a sign, only an assumption from other signs. The haematocrit (**c**) is an investigation not a sign and pain (**d**) would in fact disappear if the splenic capsule ruptured and the shock would then become very marked.

17.5 **d** Allergic response is quite common and seems to be mainly due to the subgrouping within the donated blood rather than to the main grouping. Option **a** describes what might happen if there is a mismatch. A mild reaction will often respond to an injection of chlorpheniramine maleate (Piriton).

17.6 **d** As with appendicectomy there is very little loss to or change in the overall functioning of the body with the loss of the spleen.

17.7 **b** The underlying principle of wound care is to reduce infection to the minimum. Options **a**, **c** and **d** would also occur if the nurse attempted to draw the knot through the skin.

17.8 **c** 250 mg × 6 doses × 5 days = 250 × 30 = 7500 mg or 7.5 g. Benzylpenicillin is derived from a different fungal mould (**a**) and is specific to a narrow range of bacteria. Options **b** and **d** are irrelevant as regards the dose. There is a risk of 10% of the United Kingdom population being allergic to ampicillin.

17.9 **d** The patient will have a physiotherapist at the football club who will concentrate on strengthening the muscles which have been incised mainly to avoid an incisional hernia. Joe's antibiotics (**a**) will have been completed before discharge from hospital, i.e., a five day course but he remained 7 days in hospital. Option **b** is irrelevant and **c** is a personal decision which should not be based on the surgical history.

17.10 **c** Options **a**, **b** and **d** are more effectively organized by other parts and systems of the body. Erythrocytes (**a**) are produced at the extremities of long bones and options **b** and **d** by the lymphatic system.

18 Hydrocephalus

ANSWER SHEET

18.1 a For a whole variety of reasons including options **b** and **d** the design of paediatric units must include isolation cubicles to care for infants under the age of 13 months. This is recommended by the Department of Health.

18.2 c The flow of cerebrospinal fluid is obstructed, this distends the ventricles within the brain which in turn displaces and distends the sutures and fontanelles of the cranial bones. The cranial circumference is measured at birth and should not increase in diameter. After several weeks or months the cranial bones are visually noticeable to be disproportionately larger than the facial bones. Options **a** and **d** occur once the pressure intrudes into the brain substance. Convulsions (**b**) are a sign of very many childhood diseases.

18.3 c The obstruction to the flow of cerebrospinal fluid may occur at the base of the fourth ventricle (**d**). However, it may also occur along the Aqueduct of Sylvius or within the third ventricle. Options **a** and **b** are the results of obstruction and not the cause.

18.4 a The valve itself is secured into the lateral ventricle via a burr hole operation through the bones of the skull. The tubing attached to the valve is taken via the subcutaneous tissues of the neck and threaded into the venous system until it comes to rest in the right atrium where excess cerebrospinal fluid will drain. The apparatus includes a one-way valve which automatically closes when the pressures in the right atrium are altered by coughing, swallowing, crying or other activities requiring strenuous effort.

18.5 c Also known as the Abducens nerve which supplies the lateral rectus muscle of the eye. The trigeminal nerve (**a**) is also known as the fifth cranial nerve and has branches to the muscles of the head and face, particularly those muscles dealing with chewing. The third cranial nerve (**b**) is the oculomotor nerve and supplies the ciliary and iris muscles which regulate the size and diameter of the pupil of the eye. The twelfth cranial nerve (**d**) or the hypoglossal nerve supplies the muscles of the tongue particularly those dealing with movement.

18.6 a Option **b** is false, in fact, patients given halothane anaesthesia often require analgesia on recovery from surgery. Rapid hypotension (**c**) would be a dangerous technique and, if required, is carried out very slowly. Most anaesthetics would give a fairly rapid (**d**) not a slow induction.

18.7 a Paracetamol may in fact cause vomiting (**b**), nausea (**c**) and (**d**). Its anti-inflammatory properties, however, are minimal.

18.8 a Option **b** would be a very difficult visual observation to make. Since the tip of the tubing is resting in the right atria there may be some cardiac irritation which, apart from pulse recordings, would have to be indicated by a cardiac monitor. Option **d** is possible but is more likely to be due to the feeding technique rather than the valve or its attached tubing.

18.9 d Option **a** is false information. Spontaneous recovery (**b**) of cerebrospinal fluid flow is possible but it would be inadvisable to offer this information in case it created false hopes; obviously the valve would be removed in such an instance. It is not common practice to replace the valve (**c**) at regular intervals.

18.10 d See also answer 18.4.

19 Appendicitis

ANSWER SHEET

19.1 d The pain of appendicitis is vague until it settles in the right iliac fossa and radiates to the centre of the abdomen. On pressure release at McBurney's point (right iliac fossa) there is an acute pain which is almost diagnostic of appendicitis, although this can only be proved at surgery.

19.2 c Reference to any anatomy text will clarify the correct answer.

19.3 b Options **c** and **d** are incorrect statements. If the appendix is positioned retrocaecally or subcaecally it may prove difficult for the surgeon to mobilize the inflamed structure, but it would not necessarily make its removal difficult, once it is mobilized.

19.4 b $125+(62.5 \times 10)=750$ mg.

19.5 a When the appendix lumen becomes obstructed by a faecalith, any potentially pathogenic micro-organism rapidly multiplies to form pus and suppuration. In the process the mucosa becomes inflamed. Should the single appendicular artery and vein be obstructed in their bloodflow, necrosis and gangrene can occur unless there is surgical intervention. Should the appendix rupture the infected contents escape into the peritoneal cavity causing an inflammation of the peritoneum.

19.6 a While accepting some minor changes in the temperature and pulse the nurse needs to be vigilant in the changing nature of the pain of appendicitis. The abdominal pain diminishes but the abdominal muscles increase in rigidity, frequently referred to as muscle guarding, when the appendicitis progresses to a rupture and peritonitis.

19.7 c At the time of wakening, the unfamiliar environment is the greatest psychological threat to children in hospital, the anxiety being reduced by the presence of the central figure of love and security. Options **b** and **d** are incorrect statements for a boy aged 4. Familiarity (**a**), in this context, is true but it is a general statement not referring to anaesthesia. The mother–child relationship is temporarily discontinued by hospitalization.

19.8 d Option **c** is usually noted in pyloric stenosis, while options **b** then **a** usually follow option **d**.

19.9 d See also answer 19.1.

19.10 a Second intention (**d**), as the term implies, is that healing is a secondary consideration and such a wound would have a drain secured so that excess exudate can escape to the surface. After the wound has drained satisfactorily and the drain removed, it will heal by granulation (**b**). Granulation is the healing of a wound from the base upwards and the wound edges are not approximated by sutures. A primary suture usually refers to the suture securing the drain to the wound edges which is the first suture to be removed before the wound drain can be shortened.

20 Cholecystectomy

ANSWER SHEET

20.1 b The right and left hepatic ducts (**c**) are within the liver and convey bile towards the cystic duct (**a**), both being unlikely sites for gallstones. Gallstones lying in the gallbladder (**d**) would have to be extremely large before they could actually block the excretion of bile.

20.2 b Calomel lotion (**a**) was formerly used as a purgative, camphor oil (**c**) was formerly used as a carminative and cetrimide solution (**d**) is an antiseptic lotion.

20.3 a The hormones cholecystokinin and pancreozymin are secreted from cells in the gastric mucosa in the presence of fat in the stomach. The effect of the hormones is to contract the gallbladder so that bile is ejected into the duodenum and to increase the secretion of pancreatic juice which is rich in digestive enzymes.

20.4 b The liver can only synthesize prothrombin and fibrinogen when there is an adequate amount of vitamin K in the blood. Prothrombin and fibrinogen are plasma proteins and both are essential for the natural coagulation of blood. Vitamin K is fat-soluble and therefore requires bile for its absorption from the intestine. If there is any suggestion of biliary obstruction there may be a tendency towards vitamin K deficiency which is corrected by giving vitamin K by injection before and after surgery to reduce any tendency towards haemorrhage.

20.5 b The gallbladder receives approximately 120 ml of bile from the liver in 24 hours. It concentrates this volume down, however, to between 50 and 60 ml by absorption of water and the addition of mucin.

20.6 c Vitamin K will not be absorbed unless bile is present, particularly bile salts. Serum bilirubin (**a**) is the end result of bile absorption, cholecystokinin (**b**) is a gastric hormone, and bile pigments (**d**) are derived from broken down blood cells. See also answer 20.4.

20.7 c Many surgical procedures result in a temporary oedema of the tissues surrounding the operation site. In the initial postoperative period such an oedema could occlude the patency of the common bile duct. Option **a** is true but is not a primary reason. It is important to measure any bile (**b**) drained via the T tube but more difficult to measure any exudate from the wound itself. Option **d** is a remote possibility if the stones have been removed.

20.8 b Since the operation site, the upper right abdomen immediately below the diaphragm, has a complex wound drainage, the breathing will not only be painful but also very shallow giving rise to the risk of chest infection. The hepatic flexure of the large intestine will most probably have been mobilized during surgery leading to a paralytic ileus hence abdominal distension. Hypotension (**a**) would be expected in the early postoperative phase being the result of shock and anaesthesia and is not a complication. Retention of urine (**c**) is common following all abdominal operations but not specifically a cholecystectomy, and a burst abdomen (**d**) is a remote possibility on a wound where there is a drain.

20.9 c The T tube is a rigid structure and its wide diameter ensures that it does not become blocked. In the healing process the volume of bile being drained should reduce in volume in each successive day, indicating that the bile duct is patent. A cholangiogram has nothing to do with proving healing (**b**) of the operation site or with the serum bilirubin (**d**).

20.10 c Options **a**, **b** and **d**, if they occur, would do so in the postoperative period while the patient was in hospital.

Orthopaedic Case Histories

21 Fracture of the Radius and Ulna

ANSWER SHEET

21.1 a Bennett's fracture (b) is a break in the first metacarpal bone usually combined with a subluxation. Pott's Fracture (c) is diagnosed according to degree: first degree is a break of the lateral malleolus only; in a second degree break both malleoli are broken with a displaced talus bone and third degree means that the talus bone is displaced backwards, both malleoli and the tibia are broken. Smith's fracture (d) is a fracture of the lower end of the radius with a backward displacement of the broken bone fragment and is often referred to as a reverse Colles' fracture.

21.2 a The general rule for undressing the injured patient is to undress from the healthy side and to dress from the injured side to minimize the amount of handling and movement of the patient.

21.3 d No artificial means are required to aid the drying of plaster of Paris as the heat emitted from the plaster is a chemical interaction between the gypsum and water. Plaster casts should have thoroughly dried within 24 hours of their being applied and during the drying phase should be well supported on a firm base.

21.4 c Unequal and dilated pupils imply that the intracranial pressure is abnormal, i.e., raised, and that sensory impulses from the circular muscles of the iris are not being relayed to the retinal coat and back along the optic nerve to the occipital lobe.

21.5 d Windows (a) should only be cut into plaster casts when there is a wound which requires daily dressings and/or observations. Bivalving (b) of the cast is done when there is severe swelling of the affected limb. Active physiotherapy (c) would not relieve the itching sensation. If the itching and irritation become unbearable the cast should be removed, the limb checked, and a new cast applied.

21.6 c An increased intensity of bright light causes the radiating and circular muscles of the iris to constrict making the pupils of the eye pinpoint. When the lens has accommodated to the light the muscles of the iris will relax and the pupil dilates to allow the light to enter and reach the retina.

21.7 c A long bone is defined as having a shaft and two extremities.

21.8 c The initial reaction of many sensible and caring parents when an accident occurs is to feel they are not in control of their children and have not done enough to protect their children from everyday hazards. This creates a feeling of guilt even when they have, in fact, done all that is possible. The emotions of anger, despair and hysteria may follow. An understanding of emotional response will help with communication and the problems inherent in dealing with distraught relatives.

21.9 b Polythene protective sheeting (**a**) is most useful advice but not the most important, a soiled cast can always be replaced. Option **c** is most probable especially if the cast is very heavy. Option **d** is irrelevant since the cast will be dry before hospital discharge. Flexion and extension of the fingers will reduce any tendency to swelling and keep the muscles of the arm in good tone.

21.10 b Home accidents (**a**) are highest in the under 6 years age group. School playgrounds (**c**) have a relatively low rate of accidents especially when the children are supervised. Many of the accidents arising in school playgrounds arise from badly designed outdoor equipment. Rivers and waterways (**d**) still claim a great number of lives but not as many as the main roadways.

22 Rheumatoid Arthritis

ANSWER SHEET

22.1 c The peripheral small joints are symmetrically affected by the acute inflammation and should be completely 'rested' during an acute attack. When the ESR has returned to within normal levels then options **a** and **b** are valid. Wheelchair dependency (**d**) is not a practical suggestion since the joints of the hands would not be able to negotiate the wheels unless an electrically operated chair were available.

22.2 d The pain of acute rheumatoid arthritis is diurnal in nature being extremely bad on awakening and becoming tolerable towards the evening. Part of the pain is due to stiffness of the joints and this is combined with the inflammation of the joint. This diurnal nature of the pain is a useful guideline as to when anti-inflammatory drugs should be timed to give the maximum of relief.

22.3 b See also answer 22.1.

22.4 b Acetylsalicylate acid (Aspirin) remains one of the most effective drugs in the treatment of rheumatoid arthritis.

22.5 d The rheumatoid factor, an antiglobulin in the sera of affected patients is measurably present in 80% of those who suffer from the disease. However, it is also present in the sera of many elderly patients who do not suffer from rheumatoid arthritis and quite commonly found in those with hepatic and other diseases.

22.6 d Option **a** is the normal ESR for male patients and option **b** for female patients, while option **c** is the raised ESR to be expected in male patients with an inflammatory disorder.

22.7 c The inflammatory process increases the viscosity of the membranes of the erythrocytes tending to make them form 'rouleaux' and thus becoming heavier. It is not an infective pathology so the leucocyte level while active may not necessarily be raised. There are over 17 coagulation factors which combine in a cascade when coagulation is required, there is no evidence that all the factors become viscous during an inflammatory process.

22.8 a Prednisolone is predominantly an anti-inflammatory agent derived from the steroid group of drugs, many of the steroids are also mildly antiallergic.

22.9 a $(50 \times 10)+(25 \times 7)+(15 \times 3)=500+175+45=0.720$ g.

22.10 c Although rheumatoid arthritis is a crippling and disabling disease it is not on the official list of chronic illnesses exempt from current prescription charges. Three avenues are possible to reduce the prescription cost to this patient. If the patient can prove she is receiving Supplementary Benefit, Family Income Supplement or if her general practitioner declares that she is so handicapped that she cannot go out unless accompanied by another person this may qualify her for exemption of payment for prescribed drugs.

23 Below Knee Amputation

ANSWER SHEET

23.1 c This is one form of a group of diseases which cause intermittent claudication. Homans' sign refers to pain in the calf muscle on flexion of the foot and is indicative of deep vein thrombosis. Raynaud's disease (**b**) is similar in nature to Buerger's disease but affects the arteries of the hands. Varicose veins (**d**) do not give rise to the symptoms of peripheral arterial disease.

23.2 c Alcohol (**a**) in this instance in minimal and moderate amounts actually helps to dilate blood vessels. His slight overweight (**b**) would not make a radical difference to the surgery or its prognosis. Elasticated hosiery (**d**) is a comforting palliative measure but would not alter the prognosis or the long-term outlook.

23.3 c A great number of amputees suffer phantom pain for a much longer period than the actual stump pain. Often phantom pain delays expected progress and therefore some emphasis before surgery helps the patient to understand and cope with the postoperative difficulties.

23.4 c The time period of 24 hours is too short for either options **a** or **b**. Ambulation will not influence the problem of loss of body image (**d**) although it may increase the patient's awareness of the adaptations now required.

23.5 d Any major operation carries with it the 'immediate' danger of shock and the observations of pulse and blood pressure during the initial postoperative phase are vital to detect its presence.

23.6 b Reactionary haemorrhage if it occurs is due to the blood pressure returning to normal levels after the anaesthesia has worn off. Primary haemorrhage (**b**) occurs at the time of injury or surgery, secondary haemorrhage (**c**) occurs 7–10 days after injury or surgery and is due to infection. Accidental haemorrhage (**a**) is not a phrase in common use.

23.7 d It is impossible to take the body weight on the shoulders (**a**); any weight applied into the axillae causes indirect pressure on the brachial and radial nerves (**b**) and the wrists quickly become painful if they sustain any body weight (**c**).

23.8 d The flexion deformity occurs at the groin crease with the stump tending to flex upwards unless it is restrained in the initial phase by a roller towel held firm to the mattress surface by sandbags. After any wound drains have been removed the patient is gently placed lying on his stomach. This position will push the flexed stump into extension thus countering any tendency to a permanent flexion deformity.

23.9 a Cleanliness and dryness (**b**) of the stump applies at all times not just for the stage of recovery mentioned. Although the prosthesis is a temporary one (**c**) it should fit equally as well as the permanent artificial limb and therefore the crutches would not be encouraged. Balance (**d**) is not the main problem since the aims of physiotherapy would be to attain good balance for the fitting and wearing of the temporary prosthesis. More of a problem will be the skin excoriation to be expected from the rubbing onto the stump, hence the need to wear a stump bandage.

23.10 c The rehabilitation officer will have all the reports and recommendations of the physiotherapist, medical social worker and surgeon and will also know of the current employment situations within the building industry.

24 Midshaft Femur Fracture

ANSWER SHEET

24.1 d An oblique fracture can be classified as being of the 'simple' type in which there is no wound present; this excludes options **a** and **d**. Manual manipulation equates with 'open reduction under general anaesthetic' when the bone ends are manipulated to realignment using X-rays as the guideline. This is not a surgical (**c**) procedure.

24.2 d The greatest emphasis must be given to the correct fitting and padding of the leather ring of the Thomas splint. If it is fitted too loosely there will be inadequate traction, if too tight, it causes painful pressure in the groin. Options **c**, then **b** and finally **a** would be the priorities.

24.3 c Pressure as opposed to traction will be greatest at the groin from the ring of the Thomas splint. The ischial tuberosity (**a**) should be free of the splint. The sacrum is subject to pressure not from the splint but as a consequence of being confined to bed. The internal malleolus (**d**) will be subject to pressure from the skin extension but it should be padded as protection from the bars of the splint.

24.4 a Elevating the foot of the bed not only relieves pressure at the groin but also assists in reducing any tissue swelling around the fracture site. The pull or traction is provided by the splint, countertraction (**b**) is provided by the upper half of the body. Abduction (**c**) or external rotation of the foot is desirable but not brought about by elevating the foot of the bed and the same is true of option **b**.

24.5 b With qualified supervision options **a**, **c** and **d** are well within the scope of a trained nurse. However, medial rotation implies the limb must be realigned so that the knee points directly upwards and this requires an adjustment of the complete splint and its apparatus.

24.6 a The healing time of bone is not influenced by sliding or fixed traction. Such time is reduced with the use of orthopaedic pins, plates and screws when the preliminary stages of healing are bypassed. Options **c** and **d** are not necessarily true.

24.7 b A windlass is a wedge of wood which when twisted between the traction cords takes up any slack. The twist is made between the end of the Thomas splint and the base of the skin extension kit. The weights (**a** and **c**) should **not** be altered otherwise they put at risk the union between the fractured bone ends and if weights are to be altered the surgeon's permission must be obtained. Elevation of the foot of the bed (**c**) will release pressure at the groin.

24.8 b The lateral aspect of a limb is its outer aspect so to avoid any possible friction with the healthy limb the pins are never fixed on the midline. Option **a** is true but has no bearing on the question asked. Options **c** and **d** are irrelevant.

24.9 a See also answer 24.4.

24.10 c The nutrient artery and its branches are usually breached at the time of fracture causing a haematoma around the broken bone ends, therefore, since there is very limited space haemorrhage into the bone is limited. The sequence of healing is option **c**, **a**, **b** and finally **d**.

25 Meniscectomy

ANSWER SHEET

25.1 b Massage (**c**) and the alcohol rub (**d**) may help if the knee has become locked, but would not control the joint effusion which commonly arises within 24 hours of an injury. A hot compress (**a**) increases the risk of joint effusion because it dilates the local blood vessels.

25.2 a The twisting movement of the knee is caused usually by a violent rotational force against a flexed knee while the foot is fixed to the ground. In normal activity the knee cannot rotate (**b** and **c**), nor can the knee flex and extend at the same time (**d**).

25.3 c An assessment is made to determine the degree of muscle wasting of the affected leg and the limitation of the movements of flexion and extension brought about by the torn meniscus. Aspiration of joint fluid (**d**) is a possibility but would not influence the actual planned operation. Antibiotics (**a**) and grouping and crossmatching of blood (**b**) are possible but slightly unusual in this operation.

25.4 d The affected limb is maintained in an extended position on the flat surface of a firm mattress, i.e., at 0°. Flexion (**a** and **c**) would lead to a great deal of pain if not also deformity, while extension at a 90° angle would require some form of traction to raise the leg free from the mattress surface.

25.5 b A Robert Jones bandage uses three crepe bandages, each bandage being separated by a layer of cotton wool. This is firmly applied from midthigh to midcalf and acts as a splint keeping the joint immobilized. It minimizes rather than prevents (**c**) joint effusion. The effect of surgery will be to give a more stable joint (**a**) and while the bandage has an indirect effect on the local circulation it has very little to do with maintaining (**d**) the blood supply.

25.6 **c** The quadricep group of muscles consisting of the rectus femoris, vastus intermedius, vastus medialis, and vastus lateralus are responsible for both extension and flexion of the leg and require strengthening to compensate for the removal of the meniscus. The gluteal muscle group (**d**) abducts the thigh and the hamstring group (**a**) extends the thigh but only flexes the knee joint. The gastrocnemius or calf muscle extends the foot and flexes the lower leg.

25.7 **b** X-ray, palpatory examination and the strength of the quadricep muscle group determine when the risk of joint effusion is over. If the physiotherapy regimen has been faithfully followed there should be minimal joint stiffness (**a**). The sutures (**c**) will be removed between the 7th and 10th postoperative day and have no relevance to weightbearing. The infection risk (**d**) in meniscectomy is of a low incidence.

25.8 **b** The effort required to raise a straight leg with a weight placed over the foot contracts, not extends, (**a**) the muscles. While in a state of contraction during leg-raising exercises the knee joint can be felt to extend. The knee joint itself cannot be contracted (**c**) only the muscles above and below. Muscles either contract or relax, it is joints which flex (**d**) or extend as the result.

25.9 **d** The lateral, medial and cruciate ligaments combine to limit the joint movement to flexion and extension thereby giving the joint its stability. Only the lateral and medial ligaments are referred to as menisci, not the cruciate ligament (**b**) which is at the back of the knee joint.

25.10 **b** The aim of the operation is to return the patient to a full and active life. After a further 4 weeks of remedial physiotherapy and an outpatients check up the patient should be able to resume all his former activities.

26 Laminectomy

ANSWER SHEET

26.1 **c** The traction used would need to be bilateral to exert an equal pull on either side of the vertebral column. Skeletal traction (**a**) is a direct pull on a given bone, Hamilton–Russell traction (**b**) is used for fractures of the lower third of the femur, upper third of the tibia and as a temporary traction in fractured neck of femur in the elderly. Fixed skin traction, e.g., Thomas splint (**d**) is inappropriate therapy for vertebral lesions.

26.2 **c** The lumbar vertebra takes the greatest mechanical stress when a person is lifting, pulling or pushing any object as it is the central fulcrum of the longitudinal axis which is the vertebral column.

26.3 **a** The radiopaque dye clearly outlines the spaces (theca) of the spinal cord. The dye will indicate abnormal indurations along the length of the spinal meninges which may suggest a vertebral disc lesion.

26.4 **a** Fibres of the spinothalamic tract do not cross within the spinal cord and since this is a sensory pathway the fibres give rise to pain on the right side below the level of the vertebral lesion.

26.5 **b** The nucleus pulposus is a crystalline disc lying in the centre of each intervertebral cartilage. Should this disc become displaced it causes pressure on the nerve roots entering the spinal cord. When the disc and possibly the cartilage have been removed and the vertebral bones have fused together the irritation to the nerve roots and nerve pathways should be eliminated.

26.6 **b** Arthroplasty (**a**) is the reconstruction of a diseased joint. It can be done in one of three ways; by excision of damaged tissue; by half joint replacement and by total joint replacement. Arthrectomy (**c**), taken literally, means the excision of a joint, a rare procedure. Arthrostomy (**d**) means to open into a joint.

26.7 c Spinal shock (**a**) is more obviously related to trauma and injury of the spine. Discomfort from thirst rather than dehydration (**b**) is more usual in a controlled surgical situation. There may be some localized spinal oedema (**d**) but this is quite usual to any operative site. The normal position for the male to pass urine is standing upright, so the dorsal position would inhibit normal habit.

26.8 a Gently performed, these exercises strengthen all the muscle groups of both legs and extend the knee and ankle joints which will contribute to coordination and balance once the patient is ambulant. The other options could be encouraged but in isolation would not help in the programme of mobility.

26.9 b An amphiarthrotic joint is cartilaginous, meaning it is slightly movable. The total movement of the vertebral column, however, gives extensive movements. Diarthrosis (**c**) refers to freely movable synovial joints, e.g., ball and socket joints. Synarthrosis (**a**) refers to an immovable joint such as the sutures of the skull. A condyloid joint has diarthrotic movement but refers in the main to the wrist joint.

26.10 a The spine should not be flexed during lifting eliminating options **b** and **c**. The lever action of the lumbar spine is greatly decreased when the feet are placed together (**d**) during a lift.

27 Congenital Dislocation of the Hip

ANSWER SHEET

27.1 c The evidence to date is not convincing either way, while it may be said to be familial this does not equate with a genetic (**a**) cause. There may be some relationship between virus infection and the first 12 weeks of pregnancy (**d**). A breech delivery (**b**), because of the difficulties associated with a bottom-first presentation, was thought to be a contributory factor in recent times.

27.2 b This information is derived from statistics compiled by the Registrar General of England and Wales.

27.3 a Ortolani's sign is detected when both legs are fully flexed towards the hip joints, if a clicking sound is heard it suggests that the femoral head is not secure within the rim of the acetabular cup and a possible dislocation exists. This test should be done on every baby within the first few days of life and the earlier the diagnosis the more optimistic the outlook for a complete correction.

27.4 c The thicker the nappy folds between the thighs the more the thighs are abducted, i.e., pushed away from the midline. This extra thickness and abduction will encourage the femoral head to remain within the acetabular cup.

27.5 d The approximate calculation for the fluid intake of an infant is 150 ml per kg of bodyweight per day. This volume will ensure adequate sustenance, permitting normal growth.

Therefore 150 ml × 5 kg (bodyweight) ÷ 5 feeds = 150 ml

27.6 c Being nursed in the prone position also assists in the general aim of keeping the femoral head within the acetabular cup. However, it does carry with it the risk of suffocation hence the need to keep soft surfaces, e.g., small pillows away from the infant's head.

27.7 c Although the programme of treatment covers a prolonged period, this is due to the need for further growth and development before direct therapy can be given. The earlier the treatment is planned the better the prognosis and the less likelihood of a permanent limp during childhood. See also 27.3.

27.8 c Each leg has a skin extension applied which is secured by bandaging. The cords of each skin extension are taken to a Gallows framework overhead and the legs are vertically suspended with the buttocks slightly clear of the mattress surface. This will ensure that the infant's bodyweight acts as countertraction. The head of the cot or bed should be slightly elevated to allow the child to take a visual interest in the ward environment.

27.9 d To maintain the hip reduction achieved by the vertical Gallows traction the Lorenz (frog) plaster is applied to create the widest possible abduction of the thighs, i.e., 180°. Once the cast has dried it is surprising how comfortable the child becomes in what appears to be a distressing position.

27.10 b After a few days of adjustment the child will quickly learn to adapt and enjoy play and activities within the restraint of the cast. Passive physiotherapy (**a**) is reserved for flaccid limbs or those affected by paralysis. Option **d** is undesirable in a toddler. Toilet difficulties (**c**) are overcome by shaping and cutting windows into the cast at the perineum and covering the edges of the plastercast with polythene sheeting.

28 Spinal Cord Injury

ANSWER SHEET

28.1 b In first aid the body must be positioned to allow the vertebral column to be supported in its natural contours with the patient lying flat. Some of the instances of paralysis arise not from the injury but from flexing or extending the spine after the injury worsening any minor damage to the nerve fibres.

28.2 c The 'initial' reaction would be for the muscles to contract immediately at the time of injury and in so doing act as a natural and local splint to the bones and viscera. Their contraction is sustained for quite a considerable period of time masking other signs of injury.

28.3 a A transection of spinal cord at whatever level will involve all the nerve pathways below the level of injury, this includes the sympathetic and parasympathetic nervous system.

28.4 **d** This in part also refers to muscular spasm as well as the jolt and jarring of the cord itself. There is a need to be extremely cautious in counselling the patient's relatives during this period in case the spinal shock is masking other signs of spinal cord injury.

28.5 **c** Rhizotomy involves cutting a nerve which supplies a muscle or group of muscles which are giving rise to intolerable pain, such muscles may be around or immediately above the site of injury.

28.6 **a** With prolonged bedrest there tends to be a natural increase in the deposits of calcium salts within the kidney which may, over a period of time, come to form a calculus or stone.

28.7 **d** A diaphoresis or profuse perspiration is a phenomenon of spinal cord injury which soon passes once the sympathetic (increased activity) nervous system regains its natural 'tone'.

28.8 **d** Without a nerve supply to the rectum, anal sphincters or pelvic muscles the normal advice regarding bowel habits and defaecation is rather pointless. Many paraplegic patients are taught this method of bowel evacuation if they are able to cope with the distaste of the task.

28.9 **b** The physiological response on being moved from the dorsal to the recumbent position is a shift in the blood circulation, hence fainting when the cerebral blood pressure temporarily falls.

28.10 **b** Competitive sports are universally accepted for paraplegic groups as their main outlet not only for social activity but to promote as much independence as possible within the limits of their disability. Option **a** is for future employment and is linked to **c**, who will make an assessment of possible work the patient could undertake. Option **d** only suggests two possible sports out of a very long list.

29 Fracture of the Ankle

ANSWER SHEET

29.1 **c** The time interval of 30 minutes would indicate that the ambulance had arrived promptly and the crew would have taken responsibility for any first aid given. It is not recommended to remove footwear (**b**) from those with foot injuries, since the footwear acts as a splint until the victim reaches hospital. If the footwear is left alone then it is impossible to apply a cold compress (**a**). Answer **d** is a possibility but there would need to be padding between the malleoli.

29.2 **b** If Sally is $15\frac{1}{2}$ years old then her brother will be over 16 years of age and in this situation could act as 'locus parentis'.

29.3 **a** Pott's fracture always implicates the lower third of the tibia; therefore options **a** and **c** are possible answers. Since the tibia articulates with the calcaneus, option **a** is the most correct answer. The internal malleoli (**c**) is not usually damaged on an 'inverted' foot injury. The calcaneus (**b**) is the heel bone; the fibula (**d**) is not implicated in this particular injury.

29.4 **b** It is possible to have a haematoma (**a** and **c**) and bruising (**a** and **d**) without any swelling of the surrounding tissues.

29.5 **c** The foot has a longitudinal arch which has two aspects, i.e., a medial and a lateral arch. The third arch is formed where the tarsal bones meet the metatarsal bones. The ankle has only 3 bones contributing to its structure (**a**), the carpal bones (**b**) form the wrist joint and the metatarsal bones (**d**) are independent of the phalanges being separate bones.

29.6 **b** The signs and symptoms of fractures and sprains are remarkably similar although X-ray results commonly show that sprains are more frequent than fractures. However, the sensible first aid approach would be to treat as a fracture until proved otherwise.

29.7 **b** The swelling of the ankle will resolve more quickly if the leg is slightly elevated to aid venous return. **a**, **c** and **d** would not be influenced by elevation of the limb.

29.8 **b** The temporary use of a wheelchair is a feasible proposition but it would have to be obtained from a source other than a hospital. If the heel of the plaster is reinforced (**c**) it would suggest that a walking heel was to be applied. Physiotherapy (**d**) is not possible on a casted limb, especially a lower limb.

29.9 **c** Options **a**, **b** and **d** are observations which should be made during the drying phase of the plaster cast and should have been reported and acted upon long before the patient is due for discharge from hospital.

29.10 **a** The ankle bones consist of the lower extremity of the tibia and fibula and the talus bone. The calcaneus (**b** and **d**) is the heel bone. The ankle bones articulate by hinge movement which excludes option **c** from being correct.

30 Fracture of the Patella

ANSWER SHEET

30.1 **c** The patient is on her 23rd day of a 26 day course of prednisolone. Therefore

$$(40 \text{ mg} \times 7 \text{ days}) + (30 \times 7) + (20 \times 7) + (10 \times 2) = 280 + 210 + 140 + 20 = 650 \text{ mg}$$

30.2 **d** Steroid drugs can reduce the amount of dietary calcium absorbed from the gut. Calcium is an essential mineral which lends rigidity to bone structure.

30.3 **a** Hormones produced from the adrenal cortex include hydrocortisone, corticosterone, aldosterone, some androgens and some oestrogens. They are also grouped according to their effect, glucocorticoids affect body metabolism of carbohydrates, fats and proteins. Mineral corticoids, e.g., aldosterone, affect the mineral balance of the body, especially sodium balance. Prednisolone is a synthetic derivative of an adrenal steroid and mimics a natural glucocorticoid. The adrenal medulla (**c**) secretes adrenaline.

30.4 c See also answer 30.2.

30.5 b The joint effusion will resolve slowly given a period of bedrest and immobilization. However, the bivalving of the first cast allows for the extensive swelling accompanying the joint effusion. Linear fractures (**a**) do not require realignment, bone healing (**d**) will take much longer than 10 days.

30.6 a Citrus fruits (**b**) bananas and strawberries (**c**) and tomatoes (**d**) do not contain calcium.

30.7 b Pressure and eventual damage to the brachial nerve and its branch the radial nerve will in the long term lead to wrist drop. Options **a** and **c** can be expected but are short-term reversible problems. Option **d** is irrelevant.

30.8 c Non-slip mats are dangerous to those who are dependent on crutch walking. Climbing stairs (**b**) requires supervision not direct help and this also applies to option **a**. Option **d** may be valued but is secondary to the prevention of accidents in the home.

30.9 c The stockinette should be cut several inches longer than is required so that this extra length can be reflected over the plaster edges to reduce the friction on the skin. Itching (**a**) will occur as the hair grows and also is due to epithelial shedding. Stockinette will make no difference to either options **b** or **d**.

30.10 a Before washing the limb (**c**) the dead epithelial cells should be softened and will lift easier with an application of soothing oil. After drying the limb a fine talcum powder (**b**) will relieve a great deal of the expected itching. Option **d** is irrelevant.

Geriatric Case Histories

31 Pneumonia and Head Injury

ANSWER SHEET

31.1 c This observation is vital to detect an increase in intracranial pressure. A blow to the head combined with a temporary loss of consciousness always suggests movement of the brain within its bony vault, interruption of blood and cerebrospinal fluid flow, and pressure increasing on the various ganglia in the midbrain and on the vital centres of the medulla oblongata. Prolonged raised pressure will lead to unconsciousness.

31.2 a Restlessness, agitation and disturbed behaviour can also arise from superficial bruising of the brain tissues if it is suddenly moved against the bony vault of the skull, and the observations can remain within normal limits. See also answer 31.1.

31.3 a Diplococcus (**b**) refers to those organisms which group themselves as pairs. Pneumococcus (**c**) belongs to the genus *Staphylococcus* but is a different species. Bacterium (**d**) refers to any of the large group of unicellular, vegetative micro-organisms existing in various morphological states, e.g., oval, spherical, spiral or vibrios.

31.4 a This form of therapy should dislodge the infected tenacious mucus from the base of the lungs and make it easier for the patient to expectorate the infected material. Option **c** is only possible if the patient has already cleared the lungs of infected material. Postural drainage (**b**) would help but not in the first 24 hours. Option **d** is unusual in a conscious patient.

31.5 c Two antibiotics have been prescribed which makes option **a** only half correct. Options **b** and **d** are incorrect statements.

31.6 b Norton's Scale ranges from 1–20, the lower the score the more dependent the patient is upon nursing skills and below 14 patients are regarded as being at risk. Option **a** suggests a score between 4 and 8. Options **c** and **d** are well above a score of 14.

31.7 b Option **a** is more likely to be seen in a severe pneumococcal pneumonia, while options **c** and **d** are typical of early bronchitis.

31.8 a The normal haemoglobin for females is between 11.5 and 16.4 g per 100 cm^3 (options **c** and **d**). While **b** is low it would respond to oral therapy of iron compounds.

31.9 c In a multidisciplinary approach several members of the caring team should be competent at carrying out this task, although it is a primary role belonging to the occupational therapist. However, the recommendations of the occupational therapist are acted upon by the social worker who in turn liaises with the local authority if any major structural alterations are required to the patient's home. Nurses caring for patients in their own homes should also be capable of assessing if the home environment is suitable for the type of care required.

31.10 c Following an injury coupled by pneumonia and combined with a known psychiatric illness, the depression may be triggered off once again and a psychiatric opinion would be essential in this patient's long-term interest. Physiotherapy (**a**) is normally discontinued on recovery from pneumonia; the Mogadon (**b**) certainly requires reappraisal and this would be done by the psychiatrist. Home safety (**d**) will be considered during the home assessment.

32 Hypothermia

ANSWER SHEET

32.1 c When there are no other constraints to be considered the preferred position for the patient on the verge of or in a state of unconsciousness is always the lateral position with the head placed forwards and downwards. With constant nursing supervision this should ensure a patent airway.

32.2 c The social services department, when advised, will send a representative to switch off mains services such as gas, water and electricity and check on the internal security of the house. The police are also usually advised that the property is temporarily vacated and their patrols will check on the external security at regular intervals.

32.3 a Personal property and valuables are temporarily secured in the ward safe but at the earliest opportunity these should be handed over to the unit administrator who will issue a receipt for the property and this is given to the patient.

32.4 b Cardiac output and peripheral resistance are the major factors contributing to blood pressure and are correspondingly low in hypothermia. The plasma proteins which contribute to blood viscosity and hence blood pressure are deficient in malnutrition. For this reason the blood pressure will remain low even on recovery.

32.5 b Artificial means should never be used to raise the body temperature, if attempted this will increase the peripheral temperature at the expense of the internal or core temperature of the vital organs. It is desirable to raise the temperature by 0.6°C per hour until the rectal temperature is between 36°C and 37°C. The use of duvets and sleeping bags filled with shredded tinfoil and similar ideas are most useful in **preventing** hypothermia, not in its treatment.

32.6 b Urinary secretion (**a**) is reduced in hypothermia and until the body temperature is within the normal range excretion of urine should not be expected; nor should catheterization be attempted since the infection risk is extremely high. Chest X-ray (**c**) and blood count (**d**) are not nursing measures.

32.7 b Bedbathing (**a**) would induce a peripheral vasodilation which is undesirable. The dietician (**c**) will make a valued contribution once the patient has recovered. The daughter (**d**) would have to be contacted, but only the patient knows her actual address.

32.8 b See also answer 32.5.

32.9 a Biological enzymes are inert for some time after the initial recovery from hypothermia. Anything other than cool fluids will cause nausea and vomiting.

32.10 d Iron and carbohydrates (**a**), roughage (**b**) and fats (**c**), although essential components of the diet, are secondary in promoting the health of the skin.

33 Cerebrovascular Accident

ANSWER SHEET

33.1 b Movement of **all** the limbs is vital to enhance the time interval between the occurrence of flaccid paralysis and recovery, and passive movement should be started as soon as possible. This has several advantages of preventing the loss of muscle tone, preventing possible contractures and joint stiffness and from the outset creates a positive approach within the patient.

33.2 c Hemianopia is the loss of half the visual field in one eye. Fibres from the nasal side of the right retina cross over to the left at the optic chiasma, while fibres from the temporal retina of the same eye do not cross but remain on the right side of the optic chiasma. This problem may arise temporarily if there is any disturbance or pressure to the optic pathway from the optic chiasma to the occipital lobe.

33.3 d The nurse and the physiotherapist combine to create a programme of intensive care which will restore locomotor coordination. The occupational therapist (**a**) and the speech therapist (**b**) will normally make assessments at the early stage and introduce therapy after reasonable motor coordination has been partially restored.

33·4 **b** The tone of the bladder musculature is temporarily lost when urine is drained continuously via a catheter. To regain this tone the pressures normal to the bladder are restored by permitting the bladder to retain small volumes of residual urine before removing the catheter. Even after removal the patient tends to be incontinent and can be assisted to full continence by sphincter exercises (**a**). Options **c** and **d** are not strictly relevant to the principle of restoring urinary continence.

33·5 **d** The bedside locker should be placed on the same side as the affected arm. This reminds the patient to attempt to use the affected arm whenever reaching for an article.

33·6 **b** The middle cerebral artery and its branches supply the internal capsule of the brain; within this area the motor and sensory fibres are at their closest proximity. Whether the vascular lesion is due to thrombosis, haemorrhage or an embolus the principle symptom of hemiplegia is the highest risk. The other arteries mentioned would give rise to different symptoms. The anterior cerebral artery (**a**) supplies the frontal lobe, i.e., memory, abstract thinking and logic. The posterior cerebral artery supplies in part the occipital lobe, i.e., vision. The basilar artery and its branches supply the medulla oblongata, i.e., vital centres.

33·7 **d** The example of a caring standard from a senior to a junior colleague implies emphasizing the most important priority of the given options. It is now an accepted fact that most learning is achieved in the working situation and such learning is based on the 'model' figure, i.e., the senior nurse. Teaching (**c**) of itself does not set an example of care. Feeding a helpless patient (**b**) is a one to one relationship and the senior colleague would supervise rather than help. Option **a** is not relevant to the stem.

33·8 **d** A great deal of aftercare, especially physiotherapy, is vital if the best locomotor coordination is to be achieved and this requires much persistence on the patient's part. The amount of care (**a**) is gradually decreased as the patient gains independence. Final assessment (**b**) is made by the physician. The therapy (**c**) remains within the control of the hospital physician as long as the patient remains an outpatient of which the general practitioner will be advised.

33·9 **d** Nurses should not make prognosis, this correctly belongs to the physician's role. Options **a**, **b** and **c** are therefore irrelevant to the stem.

33·10 **d** In general terms the motor and sensory pathways cross at the medulla. Descending motor pathways from the left hemisphere innervate the muscles of the right side of the body, sensory ascending pathways cross at the medulla and their impulses are received in the left hemisphere.

34 Cataract

ANSWER SHEET

34·1 **d** Light rays entering the eye are not correctly refracted as they pass through the opaque lens, therefore the rays do not reach the periphery of the retinal coat, this being proved by an investigation of perimetry.

34·2 **b** It is still not clearly understood why the crystalline quality of the lens should gradually become opaque; its gradual nature is referred to as degenerative.

34·3 **d** The power of accommodation (**c**) requires 3 qualities, increased/decreased curvature of the lens, constriction/dilation of the pupil and convergence/divergence of both eyes towards the object being focused on. See also answer 34.1.

34·4 **d** Both eyes should be clear of infection before surgery takes place. This procedure is usually carried out at the last outpatients appointment, and the results are then available on the day of admission to hospital. Options **a**, **b** and **c** are routine observations which should be done for all patients before any type of surgery.

34·5 **b** Ophthalmic day patient surgery is becoming increasingly common as surgical techniques gain in sophistication and safety. Options **c** and **d** are useful pieces of advice on being discharged from hospital. Only one eye will be covered (**a**) after a cataract removal.

34·6 **d** The lacrimal apparatus secretes a constant tearflow which washes over the cornea and conjunctiva. The tears are drained towards the back of the nose into the inferior meatus of the nasal cavity. If the tearflow is reduced or blocked the conjunctiva becomes very dry and prone to infection.

34·7 **b** The activities of swallowing (**a** and **d**) and speech (**c**), when normal, do not markedly increase intra-ocular pressure which is 2–3 kPa (18–25 mmHg). However, all the other activities do and they are a useful guide on which to base preoperative preparation and postoperative advice.

34·8 **a** The surgical technique to remove the lens is to make a very small incision into the sclera immediately above the cornea. The removal may be either intracapsular (the lens capsule is also removed) or extracapsular (the capsule is left intact).

34·9 **d** The left, not the right eye (**a**) would be covered. Sutures within the eye are soluble (**b**) and a prescription for new spectacles will be made after 6 weeks once the eye has been rested.

34·10 **c** The composition of vitreous humour can be compared to soft gelatin and it occupies that largest chamber of the eye exerting a pressure of 2–3 kPa (18–25 mmHg) which maintains the structure and shape of the eyeball.

35 Total Hip Replacement

ANSWER SHEET

35·1 **d** The acetabulum is reamed of all its degenerative membranous tissue and a prosthetic cup cemented into the acetabular cup. The femoral head is also removed and replaced by one of a range of prostheses, e.g., Austen-Moore and Thompson.

35·2 **a** Ward activities (**b**) would not be possible with such limited movement in the preoperative phase. Another patient with a similar social background (**c**) is usually unlikely, and being a depressive personality it would not be wise to introduce Mrs Gordon to someone with a similar disease (**d**).

35·3 **c** The term *degenerative* does not mean or refer to the age of the patient, only to the wearing out of tissues and a degenerative disease can occur in young people. Autoimmunity (**d**) is being researched as a possible cause but as yet there is no clear evidence that as one ages one loses self-immunity. Inflammation (**b**) within the joint occurs in rheumatoid arthritis. Infection (**a**) would cause suppuration and joint effusion and be more acute in its pathology.

35·4 **c** After surgery the patient will require good muscular tone and strength to enable her to participate fully in the exercises enabling her to stand, walk and sit, and more so if she requires a walking frame. The affected limb (**b**) will be dealt with postoperatively. Deep breathing exercises (**a**) is a normal preoperative activity. Movement of the pelvic girdle (**d**) would be painful.

35·5 **c** Specific to total hip replacement is the potential for the prosthesis to dislocate from the acetabulum. This is caused by incorrect positioning of the pelvis and lower limbs. Urinary retention (**b**) is prevented by passing a catheter into the bladder usually at the time of surgery and would help in reducing the need of toileting with bedpans. Pressure ulcers (**a**) and chest infection (**d**) must be prevented but not 'immediately' after surgery.

35.6 **b** Vacuum wound drainage bottles, e.g., Redivac, effectively drain a wound by suction created by the vacuum within the bottle. However, as with all drainage systems it must follow the law of gravity and the drainage from the wound must flow downwards below the level of the wound.

35.7 **c** The antennae on a vacuum drainage bottle are upright when there is effective suction on the wound. When the antennae are inert the vacuum within the bottle is exhausted and should be changed.

35.8 **b** Abduction means *away from the midline* of the body, so both limbs are kept apart by placing a firm wedge between the thighs. This should effectively keep the femoral head within the acetabulum. Neutrality (**a**) or the anatomical position, and adduction (**c**) both mean the legs are positioned close together. External rotation (**d**) means that the foot is turned outwards away from the body midline.

35.9 **d** The wedge referred to could be a pillow or designed as a wedge-shaped piece of sorbo material. See also answer 35.8.

35.10 **c** Both the glide chair (**a**) and the wheelchair (**b**) are counterproductive to the main aims of physiotherapy, which is to achieve good balance with an upright posture and natural walking pace. A walking stick (**d**) would be considered when physiotherapy is concluded and the support of a walking frame is no longer required.

36 Parkinson's Disease

ANSWER SHEET

36.1 **c** The nerve cells and axons originating in the substantia nigra (black substance) are located in the midbrain, these axons terminate in the caudate nucleus and the putamen. Here in these basal ganglia dopamine released by the substantia nigra acts as a neurotransmitter.

36.2 **d** Insomnia (**a** and **c**) and incontinence (**c** and **b**) may be consequences of but are not classical to Parkinson's disease.

36.3 **b** A major disadvantage of levodopa which is the amino acid precursor of dopamine is that only 5% of the oral dose effectively crosses the blood brain barrier to reach the basal ganglia. When combined with carbidopa (Sinemet) the amount of levodopa available to the brain is increased and the side effects are reduced.

36.4 **d** The first measure to deal with stiffness, tremor, and rigidity of any muscle group is to passively put them through a range of movements. This will demonstrate to those with little self-confidence that no damage or injury will result if they try themselves. Once confidence is established the nurse could then aim for options **a**, **b** and **c**.

36.5 **b** Whenever balance is unsteady and it affects both sides of the body, a two nurse escort will increase the patient's confidence when attempting to walk. Option **a** is likely to increase dependence. Remedial hydrotherapy (**d**) is likely to frighten the patient since those with muscle tremor and poor balance do not feel safe in water.

36.6 **d** In making the patient aware of her body posture using a mirror it will correct the attitude or body image the patient has of herself. Options **b** and **c** are useful in Parkinson's disease. Articles (**a**) should be so placed that they remind the patient to use the affected side or the disabled limb.

36.7 c 'Initially' the patient was reluctant to and frightened of moving, this makes options **a** and **b** more difficult to implement. Catheterization (**d**) is always a last resort because of the high incidence of infection.

36.8 b The patient is not confined to bed once drug therapy has commenced (**a**) a comforting wash would be more appropriate. A fan (**c**) is usually provided for pyrexia, not for perspiration. A deodorant (**d**) is a comforting cosmetic measure but would not reduce the problem.

36.9 b Falls as a result of muscular rigidity, tremor, and postural imbalance even when well controlled by drugs is the greatest risk and fractures are the usual result in the elderly.

36.10 d The local housing authority normally provide warden controlled shared accommodation to single elderly persons who, although suffering from a chronic illness, are independent of nursing skills but require nursing supervision.

37 Residential Care

ANSWER SHEET

37.1 a It is a relatively simple matter to check the effectiveness of both spectacles and hearing aid. If these are satisfactory then orientation to the new environment (**b**) will be easier and more certain. Options **c** and **d** are reasonable propositions until it is realized they are not effective in assessing sensory difficulties.

37.2 a The natural loss of recoil of the arterial intima leads to the hardening of the vessel, which in turn decreases the oxygenated blood supply to the brain which for some unknown reason is more obvious at night. Options **b**, **c** and **d** are all contributory factors which exacerbate the underlying condition.

37·3 c There is of course constipation (**b**) but the fluid content of the impacted faeces around the impaction escapes and soils underclothing or bedclothing. This often gives the mistaken impression that the patient is incontinent, but such instances should be investigated by digitally examining the rectum for impaction. Options **a**, **b** and **d** may all be present and individually they are sufficient evidence which warrants further investigation.

37·4 b The first and kindest measure is to soften the hard faecal matter with a small amount of warmed olive oil, this should be retained by the patient for about 20 minutes, followed by a small evacuant enema. Options **a** and **c** can then be implemented. A manual evacuation (**d**) should be the last resort only attempted if all other methods have failed.

37·5 d Normally the preferred first action would be to address the patient by name (**c**) and remind her of where she is. However, this patient is hard of hearing and visual orientation would be the quickest method of perhaps resolving her confusion. The following sequences would then be **b** followed by **a**.

37·6 d Strictly speaking the case history does not refer to sedation invalidating options **b** and **c**.

37·7 b At night and in a strange environment with a known problem of nocturnal confusion, to offer toilet facilities would reduce or remove one possible cause which might exacerbate the tendency to confusion.

37·8 c There is nothing in the history to suggest a preference for personal hobbies, or that Mrs Ferguson would benefit from occupational therapy, which is mainly used to assess and promote the use of aids to daily living. Option **d** is irrelevant.

37·9 d There are two main types of deafness, i.e., perceptive and conductive. Most elderly people suffer from the conductive type due to sclerosis of the ossicles in the middle ear which implies that sound cannot be transmitted by vibration of the inner ear.

37.10 a Cerumen or wax will muffle the sound waves penetrating the amplifier. All the other options should be noted since they are useful hints in helping the elderly to cope with the problems of using their hearing aids.

38 Rehabilitation Programme

ANSWER SHEET

38.1 c Self image in stroke patients tends to be a half image as the brain seems to ignore parts of the body affected by the paralysis. Any stimulus which involves the whole body acts as a reminder to the patient to use the affected part but this needs the reinforcement of constant verbal praise.

38.2 b Such activities, i.e., physiotherapy, occupational therapy, music therapy, meals, television, visitors, can all be used as 'whole' situations in which the patient can be subconsciously reminded of her total body image. Self-help clinics (**c**), where they exist, are part of the occupational therapy department. Evaluation (**d**) is the part of the nursing process which measures success or failure of care, but would not influence body image. See also answer 38.1.

38.3 b Options **c** and **d** are individualized items of a total programme. Option **a** while a kind thought would not offer a programme of independence or encourage the patient's self determination. See also answer 38.1.

38.4 d Common core language refers to words which are simple to pronounce, usually those with few syllables and in common usage. The simpler and shorter the word the easier it is for the patient to pronounce.

38.5 d To express something, i.e., a verbal response in this case, while the message is understood, the response is inappropriate and suggests the lesion is in the frontal lobe of the brain which collates the messages received from the temporal lobe.

38.6 a The patient hears the verbal stimulus but cannot understand it which implies a lesion in the temporal lobe since the message is not transmitted as sense to the frontal lobe.

38.7 d Incontinence should always be expected after removing a urinary catheter. The day and night pattern of expected incontinence should be charted and used to identify the most appropriate times to toilet the patient. This should be done to avoid soiling (**b**). Option **a** will do no harm but does not answer the question. Option **c** is rarely done and then only on medical instruction.

38.8 c The 7th cranial nerve is also known as the facial nerve. Its sensory branch innervates the taste buds while its motor branch supplies the facial and scalp muscles and also the salivary glands.

38.9 a Ménière's disease is a distension of the membranous labyrinth within the inner ear. While its cause is unknown it seems to be related to a disturbance of the blood supply from a possible variety of causes, e.g., trauma, infection, etc. If palliative measures to control the symptoms of vertigo, nausea, vomiting and tinnitus fail, surgical techniques may be employed. In either form of treatment hearing is sacrificed, i.e., perceptive hearing is usually unilateral in nature, affecting the 30–60 year old age group.

38.10 c The leg brace or caliper can, within a short period, become inappropriate if the patient loses weight or develops muscular wasting of the affected limb. Options **a**, **b** and **d** are all partially correct but do not offer a permanent solution to the problem.

39 Acute Monocytic Leukaemia

ANSWER SHEET

39.1 c One of the features of acute leukaemia is its remitting and relapsing nature with no promise of a permanent cure (**a**), although the remission interval has been prolonged with modern therapy. Not **all** routine blood tests (**b**) will give normal values, e.g., the haemoglobin tends to be low during and for some time after therapy. The granulocytic tissues (**d**), i.e., those of the long bones are not usually irradiated to suppress their activity.

39.2 a A monocyte (*see* diagnosis) is one of the cells derived from the granulocytic tissues, other cells in this series include the polymorphonuclear cells, i.e., basophils, neutrophils and eosinophils. Lymphocytes (**b**) may be increased in number due to infection but are not neoplastic. There is usually increased bone marrow cellularity (**c**), but this is usually proven by a bone marrow puncture to obtain a specimen of marrow. Immune responses (**d**) are low but this is a consequence of both disease and therapy rather than the cause of the disease.

39.3 c Permeability of the capillaries is a consequence of option **a** and the proliferation of monocytes. Option **b** while suspected is not a proven fact. Option **d** is a contributory factor but not a cause.

39.4 c Cytosine arabinoside antagonizes the cancer cell to pyrimidine which is an essential metabolite to its reproduction and proliferation. Daunorubicin (**a**) is a very powerful antibiotic and also depresses the activity of the granulocytic tissues in the bone marrow. Thioguanine (**b**) antagonizes the cancer cell to purine which is an essential metabolite to its reproduction and proliferation. Prednisolone (**d**) apart from being mainly anti-inflammatory also has a lympholytic activity and reduces the permeability of the capillaries.

39.5 a See also answer 39.4.

39.6 d See also answer 39.4.

39.7 c Prior to the cystometric examination both the bladder and lower colon must be empty. The bladder is then filled with opaque fluid and a series of X-rays are taken, during which the patient is requested to hold and then pass the fluid. Retained fluid, i.e., the residual volume, may indicate a problem of ureteric reflux, stress incontinence, loss of muscular tone or urethral stricture. Comparing the history to the result of the test it suggests the bladder has lost its tone and this would require permanent catheterization, which would also help to prevent secondary problems such as pressure ulcers.

39.8 b Iron deficiency anaemia reduces the viscosity of the blood giving a lower blood pressure. The heart compensates for this lower pressure by working harder but eventually this can lead to a degree of heart failure. A failing heart means a poor venous return and therefore oedema of the ankles is one of the early symptoms. Options **a** and **c** are measures to help the ankle oedema until it is clinically resolved. Antileukaemic therapy (**d**) may be involved and contribute to the anaemia.

39.9 b Altered bowel habits (**a**) should be expected **during** and after antileukaemic therapy. Options **c** and **d** are evidence of progress and would be reassuring when offered some 2 weeks after the therapy is concluded. The effects of antileukaemic drugs leave the patients exhausted for many days.

39.10 a Option **b** is the prognosis for the chronic form of leukaemia. A normal lifespan (**c**) can be offered to many children with modern therapy. A response to treatment (**d**) can never be guaranteed.

40 Terminal Illness

ANSWER SHEET

40.1 a All four emotions are quite common to those who are terminally ill. Their degree of intensity and time overlap varies from one patient to another. The psychological approach of the caring team could be influenced by an understanding of the emotional responses of the patient.

40.2 b The impending absence of body image is also an alteration to existing self concept and induces extreme psychological trauma which is an overt hostility or anger against those around the patient at the time of the emotional experience.

40.3 c Denial can take many forms, i.e., spiritual denial, refusing against better judgement to put one's affairs in order, and refusing to cooperate with those best able to help are only a few examples.

40.4 c The professional judgement of the nurse is the best barometer of when the patient should have visitors. The nurse will know when treatments are due, examinations performed, investigations made, etc., and this can be balanced against the known pattern of the patient's rest needs.

40.5 d Procaine (**a**) is a local anaesthetic used for topical purposes. Sucrose (**b**) is unnecessary if honey is already added. Ethyl alcohol (**c**) is used mostly for topical or industrial purposes.

40.6 c The physician is the only person who could offer an accurate prognosis of the time of probable death. If asked by the patient the others mentioned could be encouraging without making any commitment.

40.7 d Physicians prefer to counsel only the next-of-kin to avoid any breach of the patient's confidences. Option **b** would be telling a lie and option **c** is unprofessional since it avoids a positive action.

40.8 **b** Cachexia is an example of tissue wasting when catabolism exceeds anabolism resulting in a negative nitrogen balance.

40.9 **c** Cardiac dyspnoea (**b** and **d**) accompanies cardiac and pulmonary congestion. Rapid respirations (**a**) are unlikely since the respirations typical of Cheyne–Stokes are paroxysmal and sighing in nature.

40.10 **b** A first reaction would be to allow the nurse those few minutes privacy to collect and calm herself or himself before resuming any duties. At a later time a cup of tea with sympathy is greatly appreciated. One way of junior colleagues working through their anguish is to help with last offices. Correctly carried out this allows the nurse the opportunity of offering a final farewell to the patient of whom the nurse has become fond.